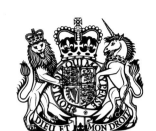

Choosing health
Making healthy choices easier

Presented to Parliament
by the Secretary of State for Health
by Command of Her Majesty

November 2004

Cm 6374

£26.00

FOREWORD

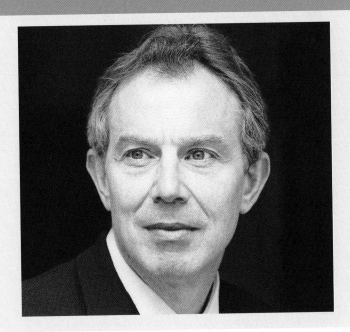

For each of us, one of the most important things in life is our own and our family's health. I believe that this concern, and the responsibility that we each take for our own health, should be the basis for improving the health of everyone across the nation.

This Government is committed to sustaining an ethos of fairness and equity – good health for everyone in England. We are already taking action throughout society to tackle the causes of ill-health and reduce inequalities. *Choosing health* sets out how we will work to provide more of the opportunities, support and information people want to enable them to choose health. It aims to inform and encourage people as individuals, and to help shape the commercial and cultural environment we live in so that it is easier to choose a healthy lifestyle.

Small changes in the choices people make can make a big difference. Taken together, these changes can lead to huge improvements in health across society. But changes need to be based on choices, not direction. We are clear that Government cannot – and should not – pretend it can 'make' the population healthy. But it can – and should – support people in making better choices for their health and the health of their families. It is for people to make the healthy

choice if they wish to. *Choosing health* sets out what this Government will do to help them.

We will build on the work of this White Paper at every level, from support for individuals right up to engaging the entire nation through events like the London 2012 Olympic Bid. I believe that *Choosing health* will be a major step in making the improvement of everyone's health everyone's concern.

Tony Blair

TONY BLAIR
PRIME MINISTER

PREFACE

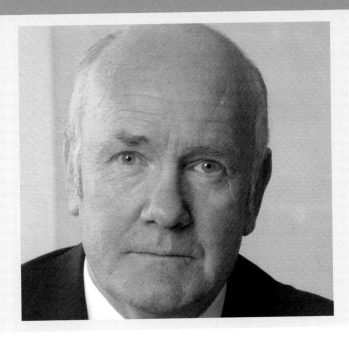

A founding principle for the NHS in 1948 was that it should improve health and prevent disease, not just provide treatment for those who are ill. Sustained investment and reform in the NHS is already ensuring faster and more personalised healthcare for patients. As the health service makes rapid progress on treating illness, the need for similar progress on improving people's health comes to the fore. We are committed to ensuring that the fundamental mission of the NHS to promote physical and mental wellbeing and prevent illness is pursued effectively in the 21st century. We need to step up the action we are taking across government and throughout society to tackle the causes of ill-health and reduce inequalities. Now is the right time to refocus the NHS as a service for health, in a way that reflects the realities of the lives of people in England today.

In recent decades, the debate about the respective roles of Government, individuals, communities, industry and others in improving health has too often become bogged down in a ritual battle between two ends of a political spectrum. On the one hand, a paternalistic state is encouraged more and more to limit individual choice, constrain personal decisions and ban action which promotes unhealthy behaviour. On the other, the Government is asked to stand back, leaving people's health to whatever the hidden hand of the market and freedom of choice produces.

The extensive consultation that informed the development of *Choosing health* has provided the opportunity to hear about what is important to people in England today. People's concerns, and ideas based on their real lives, have helped us to develop a more down-to-earth and practical approach to public health policy that will enable everyone to move on and will begin to make a real difference.

First, people told us that they want to take responsibility for their own health. They were clear that many choices they made – such as what to eat or drink, whether to smoke, whether to have sex and what contraception to use – were very personal issues. People do not want Government, or anyone else, to make these decisions for them.

Second, what they did expect was that the Government would support them in making these choices. They wanted clear and credible information, and where they wanted to make a change and found it hard to make a healthy choice they expected to be provided with support in doing so – whether directly or through changes in the environment around them – so that it is easier to 'do the right thing'.

Choosing health sets out key principles for that support. Our starting point is informed choice. People cannot be instructed to follow a healthy lifestyle in a democratic society. Health improvement depends upon people's motivation and their willingness to act on it. The Government will provide information and practical support to get people motivated and improve emotional wellbeing and access to services so that healthy choices are easier to make.

It is a fact of life that it is easier for some people to make healthy choices than others. Existing health inequalities show that opting for a healthy lifestyle is easier for some people than others. Our aim must be for **everyone** to achieve greater health and mental wellbeing by making healthier choices. That means ensuring that those people in disadvantaged areas and groups have the opportunity to live healthier lives. We will work with the many other organisations involved to coordinate effort and personalise services, tailoring them to the realities of people's lives.

While we respect individuals' rights to make their own choices, we need to respond to public concern that some people's choices can cause a nuisance and have a damaging impact on other people's health. We need to strike the right balance between allowing people to decide their own actions, while not allowing those actions to unduly inconvenience or damage the health of others.

Moreover, in the case of children there is a greater case and requirement for protection. Children need a protected environment as they learn about making lifestyle decisions that impact on their health. This is a responsibility that Government shares with parents.

These considerations, therefore, run through this White Paper: helping people to make healthier choices for themselves; protecting people's health from the actions of others; and recognising the particular needs and the importance of emotional and physical development of the young. Government cannot simply leave it up to individuals, we must work with others to provide collective support to help create an environment which promotes health. These form the basis of achieving a balance between the healthy outcomes we all want to see and the equally valued freedom to determine our own way of life that is so important in a democratic society.

Choosing health sets out a starting point for national renewal of practical and acceptable action to make a difference to the health of people in England. There is no 'magic bullet' in the strategy, because there is no quick or easy solution that is certain to work.

Some of the action set out here is substantial and will start to make a difference immediately but, in other areas, significant change will be the result of sustained action by many individuals over a number of years. This White Paper is the start, not the end of a journey. We will continue to develop ideas and action, learning from experience to help people choose health in the 21st century. It is the next step in our journey towards engaging everyone in choosing health and tackling health inequalities. We have set ambitious targets for health. By working together across society we should achieve them. The success of the strategy will be measured first in the increased number of healthy choices that individuals make, and then in the lives saved, lengthened and improved in quality.

In moving forward the public health agenda in England, we recognise that some proposals in this White Paper will have implications for other parts of the UK. We will work closely with colleagues in the devolved administrations to identify these, so that joint action can be taken where appropriate and legislative opportunities provided for the devolved administrations where new powers are created for England. In these ways we can achieve our common goal of improving the health of people throughout the UK.

JOHN REID
HEALTH SECRETARY

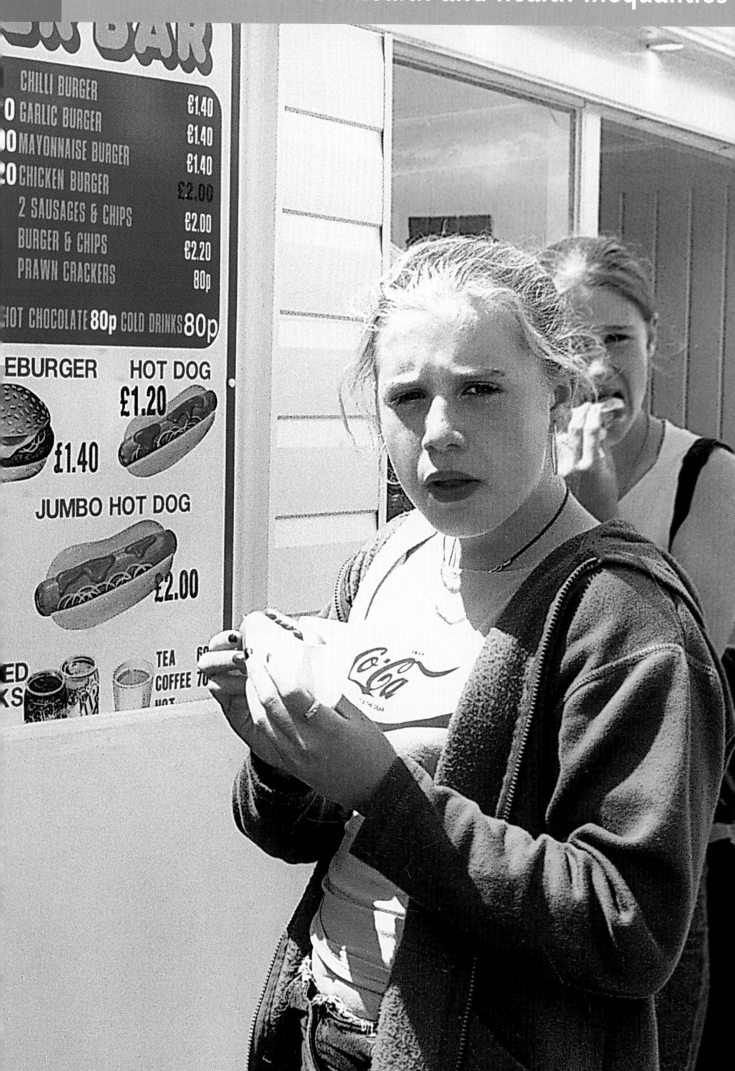

**Shift from infectious to chronic diseases as the main causes
of death over the last century**

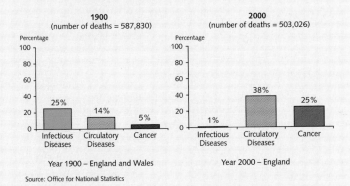

Source: Office for National Statistics

CHAPTER SUMMARY

- *Health in England has improved dramatically over the last century.*
- *New challenges have emerged and need to be tackled now if progress is to be maintained.*
- *Unfair inequalities in health have persisted and remain a key challenge.*
- *Traditional methods of improving health are becoming outdated and new approaches and new action are needed to secure progress.*
- *Consultation with the public has enabled the development of a new approach to public health, based on the reality of people's lives and the choices they make about their own health.*
- *People's lifestyle decisions are personal ones and they do not want Government to take responsibility away from them.*
- *People do want credible information and advice on lifestyle choices that impact on health and personalised support to follow through choices that they want to make but find difficult.*
- *There is support for Government to act in areas where one person's choice can affect another person's health.*
- *Society has a duty to take additional steps to protect children and young people's health.*

INTRODUCTION

1. Health is inextricably linked to the way people live their lives and the opportunities available to choose health in the communities where they live. This White Paper is about making a difference to the choices people make.

2. There have been big improvements in health and life expectancy over the last century. On the most basic measure, people are living longer than ever before. Boys born in 2004 can expect to live to the age of 76, compared with a life expectancy of 45 in 1900, and girls to 80, compared with 50 in 1900. A child born today is likely to live nine and a half years longer than a child born when the NHS was established in 1948.

3. Many factors have contributed to these improvements. Economic growth has seen rising standards of living, improved education, better nutrition and better housing for many. Many of these advances have been achieved as a result of actions taken by local authorities. There have been important advances in medicine and technology. And those advances have been made freely available to all through the NHS.

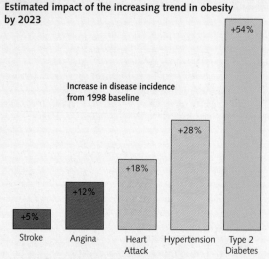

Estimated impact of the increasing trend in obesity by 2023

Increase in disease incidence from 1998 baseline

+5% Stroke
+12% Angina
+18% Heart Attack
+28% Hypertension
+54% Type 2 Diabetes

Source: Estimated effect of obesity (based on straight line extrapolation of trends) – DH-EOR (unpublished).
Note – projections should be interpreted with caution, as they assume current trends will continue unabated, which may not be realistic.

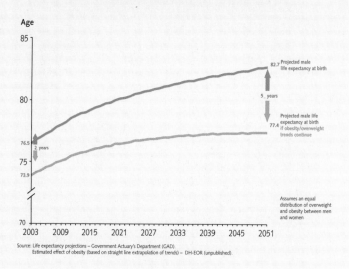

Obesity (or being overweight) is already reducing expectation of life at birth, in future the effect could be even greater

Age

82.7 Projected male life expectancy at birth

5 years

77.4 Projected male life expectancy at birth if obesity/overweight trends continue

2 years

Assumes an equal distribution of overweight and obesity between men and women

Source: Life expectancy projections – Government Actuary's Department (GAD).
Estimated effect of obesity (based on straight line extrapolation of trends) – DH-EOR (unpublished).

SUSTAINING PROGRESS

4. Future progress on this dramatic scale cannot be taken for granted. England faces new challenges to ensure that as a society we continue to benefit from longer and healthier lives. Whilst the threat of childhood death from illness is falling and the big infectious killer diseases of the last century have been eradicated or largely controlled, the relative proportion of deaths from cancers, coronary heart disease (CHD) and stroke has risen. They now account for around two-thirds of all deaths. Cancer, stroke and heart disease not only kill, but are also major causes of ill-health, preventing people from living their lives to the full and causing avoidable disability, pain and anxiety. And there are some worrying pointers for our future health:

- Smoking remains the single biggest preventable cause of ill-health and there are still over 10 million smokers in the country.
- As many as one in 10 sexually active young women may be infected with chlamydia, which can cause infertility.
- Surveys carried out since 1974 show an increase in the mental health problems experienced by young people.
- Suicide remains the commonest cause of death in men under 35.

- Around one-third of all attendances to hospital A&E departments are estimated to be alcohol-related.

HEALTH INEQUALITIES

- In a recent survey,* three out of four people reported good health in general and two out of three expect to be healthy in the future. However, here are large socio-demographic differences in health experience and expectations:
- 81% of people in higher socio-economic groups consider themselves to be in good health now, compared with 61% of people in the lowest groups
- 76% of people in the higher groups expect to be in good health in 10 years' time, compared to 53% of people in the lowest groups

  * Opinion Leader Research (OLR)

5. In addition to these emerging challenges, there are longstanding problems that need fresh approaches. We also need to focus specifically on tackling inequalities in health. Although on average we are living healthier and longer lives, health and life expectancy are not shared equally across the population. Despite overall improvements, there remain big – and in some communities increasing – differences in health between those at the top and

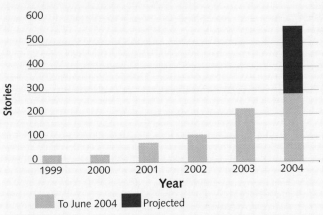

Increasing media interest: rise in stories with 'obesity' in the headline (national newspapers)

Stories (y-axis: 0, 100, 200, 300, 400, 500, 600)

Year (x-axis: 1999, 2000, 2001, 2002, 2003, 2004)

To June 2004   Projected

Source King's Fund

Note: Getting an accurate estimation of volume of stories is problematic, since stories may contain a reference to obesity but be primarily about something else. A small percentage of the data is likely to be irrelevant, but it might be safe to assume that the error rate is consistent across time.

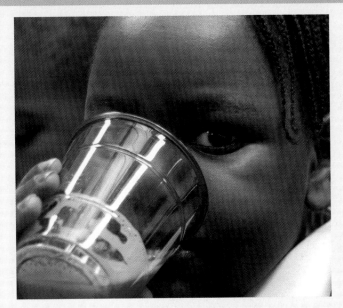

bottom ends of the social scale. Some parts of the country have the same mortality rates now as the national average in the 1950s. Mental health problems are more common in areas of deprivation.

6. Such inequalities in health are not acceptable. Our fundamental aim must be to create a society where more people, particularly those in disadvantaged groups or areas, are encouraged and enabled to make healthier choices. In order to close the gap, we must ensure that the most marginalised and excluded groups and areas in society see faster improvements in health.

7. The Government is committed to better health for everyone. We have invested record sums in the NHS. Demanding national standards for many NHS services are improving the quality of care and the end is now in sight for long waits for treatment. *The NHS Improvement Plan*[1] set out a strategy to build on that progress and provide care that is more convenient and personalised to individuals. But helping everyone to enjoy better health is about much more than faster, better and individually tailored treatment and diagnosis.

8. When the NHS was established in 1948, one of its founding principles was that it should improve health and prevent disease as well as providing treatment for those who are ill. We need to see the same systematic improvement in prevention that

we have already seen in the quality of NHS care services. Indeed, the progress made on these issues will help release capacity in the NHS to deal with deep-seated problems of health inequalities. Alongside that, we need to encourage local government, the business community and the voluntary sector to make their full contributions to promoting health and healthy choices.

PUBLIC INTEREST IN IMPROVING HEALTH

9. With new problems coming to the fore and health inequalities persisting, the time is right for new action and fresh thinking. The growing public interest in health means that there are now real opportunities to make a practical difference. Health is becoming more and more prominent in news headlines, TV programmes, magazines and everyday conversations. The media is extending the debate through coverage in the press and activities such as the BBC's *Fat Nation* and *NHS Day* and ITV's *On the Move* campaign. People's awareness of health issues and their motivation to change means that there is a much greater likelihood of achieving real progress.

10. Interest in health is being fuelled by the challenges raised in Derek Wanless's report *Securing Good Health for the Population*,[2] and the Health Select Committee's recent report on obesity.[3]

1   www.dh.gov.uk/assetRoot/04/08/45/22/04084522.pdf

2   www.hm-treasury.gov.uk/consultations_and_legislation/wanless/consult_wanless04_final_cfm

3   www.publications.parliament.uk/pa/cm200304/cm200304/cmselect/cmhealth/23/23.pdf

CONSULTATION

11. On paper, the answers can look deceptively simple – balance exercise and how much you eat, drink sensibly, practice safe sex, don't smoke. But knowing is not the same as doing. For individuals, motivation, opportunity and support all matter. To help us understand people's views about what they would find helpful – and what they would object to – the Government launched the *Choosing Health?*[4] consultation on improving people's health and the related *Choosing a Better Diet* and *Choosing Activity* consultations earlier this year.

12. We asked what could really make the difference in enabling people to choose health. What should Government do? What do individuals want to do for themselves? What support would they like from the NHS or local government? What do they expect of the food and leisure industries? What do people want for their children – and what do children and young people want for themselves? And, above all, how can we make choosing health a reality for everyone?

13. In addition, over 200 people with expertise in areas such as the food and leisure industries, employment, working with children, community development, local government and health care took part in national task groups and discussions. Together with the King's Fund and the Health Development Agency, we commissioned Opinion Leader Research (OLR) to carry out a survey of people's attitudes to health policy.[5] Further information on the consultation is at Annex A.

14. Over 150,000 people responded to the consultations directly or took part in local discussions and surveys. Most people were clear that they wanted to decide for themselves what they should do to make a difference to their own health. In our survey, 88% of respondents agreed that individuals are responsible for their own health. Health is a very personal issue. People do not want to be told how to live their lives or for Government to make decisions for them.

15. The consultation also made plain that many people do want to choose health. Building on this motivation and getting more people motivated will help improve the nation's health. This White Paper focuses on developing new demand for health.

16. But creating a demand for health is not enough on its own. If people want better health, we need to make it easier for them to do something about it. People made clear that they expect support in making these decisions, particularly the complex ones, and that sometimes they need practical help to stick to them. That is why this White Paper sets out action to help make healthier choices easier by providing better information, encouragement, help, support and services so that people know what to

4   www.dh.gov.uk/assetRoot/04/07/58/52/04075852.pdf
5   Opinion Leader Research. www.kingsfund.org.uk/pdf/publicattitudesreport.pdf

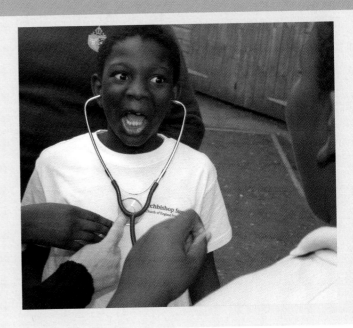

do and why, and make healthier choices that can be sustained in the longer term.

17. Healthy choices are often difficult for anyone to make, but where people do not feel in control of their environment or their personal circumstances, the task can be more challenging. People who are disabled or suffer from mental ill-health, stretched for money, out of work, poorly qualified, or who live in inadequate or temporary accommodation or in an area of high crime, are likely to experience less control over their lives than others and are often are pressed to cope with immediate priorities. They are often less likely to think about the consequences of everyday choices about diet, exercise, smoking and sexual behaviour on their long-term health, or to take up the childhood immunisation and health screening programmes that provide protection against diseases that can kill or cause serious long-term ill-health. People are more likely to take more control over their own health if they have more control over their lives.

Survey showing external factors and individual control

In a recent survey,* 46% of respondents agreed that there are too many factors outside of individual control to hold people responsible for their own health. Differences in responses for different groups suggest that people in lower socio-economic, socially excluded or black and minority ethnic groups may see health as being further beyond their individual control than others do.

* OLR

18. Health protection is a key element in public health action. There are a range of environmental hazards that national and local government tackle to protect health, but this White Paper largely focuses on the key issues, where we can make a difference by supporting individuals to make healthy choices in the communities where they live. To do that we need to work in ways that take account of the realities of people's lives, particularly those people who are relatively disadvantaged. Success here is critical in tackling health inequalities.

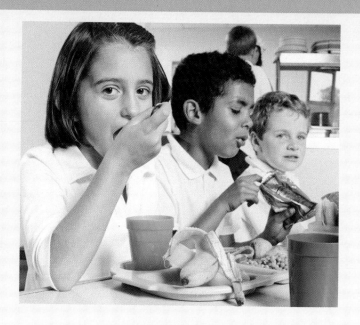

19. The response to consultation and wider research suggests that Government is expected – and trusted – to act on inequalities and on wider issues that impact on society. While these are not felt to be issues for Government alone, there is a strong role for Government in promoting social justice and tackling the wider causes of ill-health and inequality in health. Government is already acting in a number of areas, including social exclusion, neighbourhood renewal and childhood poverty.

Ethnic deprivation by locality
67% of people from ethnic minority backgrounds live in the 88 deprived areas which receive neighbourhood renewal funds compared with 40% of the total population of England.

Survey tackling poverty
In a recent survey, two-thirds of respondents agreed that tackling poverty would be the most effective means of preventing disease and improving health. People in the lowest socio-economic groups (67%) and the socially excluded (71%) are more likely to agree than people in the higher socio-economic groups.

20. People also look to Government to respond to inequalities through policy design and implementation. *Choosing health* sets out further action to target investment where it is most needed. Many of the initiatives in this White Paper will be targeted first at communities and groups where opportunities to choose health are least well-developed and most progress is needed.[6] And there is also a strong focus on building on the partnerships that already exist in communities and across government to tackle inequalities.

PRINCIPLES FOR ACHIEVING CHANGE
21. Derek Wanless's report on *Securing Good Health for the Whole Population*[7] outlined the benefits for us all if we succeed in achieving a society more fully engaged in health. The prizes are longer, healthier lives for all, fewer working days lost and reductions in pressure on healthcare in the future. He made clear that a step change is needed in the way we address health issues and tackle health inequalities and that 'more of the same' would be insufficient to deliver that change. New thinking and practical action was needed. Too often in the past we have devoted too much time and energy to analysing the problems and not enough to developing and delivering practical solutions that connect with real lives.

---

6 Although all primary care trusts are expected to tackle inequalities in health within their local populations, it is especially important to make faster progress on a larger scale in the 20% of PCTs with the worst health and deprivation indicators.

7 www.hm-treasury.gov.uk/consultations_and_legislation/wanless/consult_wanless04_final.cfm

> "I am an asthmatic and as such have problems with my breathing anyway and find nothing worse than a smoker who ignores the rules. I understand that people have the right to smoke or not, but the moment I have to breathe in their smoke they are infringing upon my rights to clean air."
>
> Consultation respondent

22. The new problems that have emerged and the old problems that have persisted are the cumulative results of thousands of choices by millions of people over decades that impact on health. So a step change in health improvement will involve millions of people making different choices about the things they do in everyday life which impact on their health. People want and are ready for change. But old solutions have not provided the impetus. We believe the right approach is to empower people, support people when they want support and to foster environments in which healthy choices are easier. The action to deliver this is underpinned by three principles.

23. While people want to make their own health decisions, they do expect the Government to help by creating the right environment. Therefore supporting informed choice for all is the first principle on which this White Paper is built. But we need to exercise a special responsibility for children who are too young to make informed choices themselves.

24. Three-quarters of respondents in the Opinion Leader Research (OLR) survey agreed that the Government should prevent people from doing things that put the health of others at risk. So we also need special arrangements for those cases where one person's choice may cause harm or nuisance to another, such as exposure to second-hand smoke. We need to balance rights and responsibilities, in ways that protect health.

25. The second key principle is the personalisation of support to make healthy choices. This will be crucial in helping to reduce health inequalities. It means building information, support and services around people's lives and ensuring that they have equal access to them.

26. Finally, people understand that improving health choices often involves many players, including themselves. Many of the responses to the consultation commented on the need for more effective working together to deal with all the factors that interact to determine health. So, working in partnership to make health everybody's business is the third principle. Local government, advertisers, industry and retailers, the NHS and other public bodies, the voluntary and community sector, communities, employers and the media all have a role. Health needs are complex and real lives do not fit neatly into the boundaries of individual organisations or government departments or organisations. So people look to the Government to lead, coordinate and promote partnership working, in support of individuals and communities.

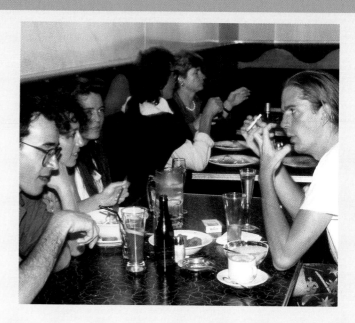

'Young people need to be specifically helped to develop the ability to: recognise and resist pressure so that they can delay intercourse until they are ready for it; develop healthy relationships; and negotiate and practise safer sex.'

Brook Advisory Centres

MAKING IT HAPPEN

27. The Government has already signalled its commitment to better health. We have included targets to improve people's chances for better health and reduce inequalities in the Public Service Agreement (PSA) framework,[8] which drives forward the Government's highest priorities and ambitions for public service delivery. Action on health will occur across government – for example, the Office of the Deputy Prime Minister leads on a Government target to tackle social exclusion and deliver neighbourhood renewal to deliver measurable improvements, including narrowing the health inequalities gap, by 2010.

CONCLUSION

28. This White Paper is the start, not the end, of a journey. We will continue to develop ideas and action, learning from experience to help people choose health in the 21st century. It is the next step in our journey towards engaging everyone in choosing health and tackling health inequalities. We have set ambitious targets for health. By working together across society we should achieve them.

---

8   www.hm-treasury.gov.uk/spending_review/spend_sr04/spend_sr04_index.cfm

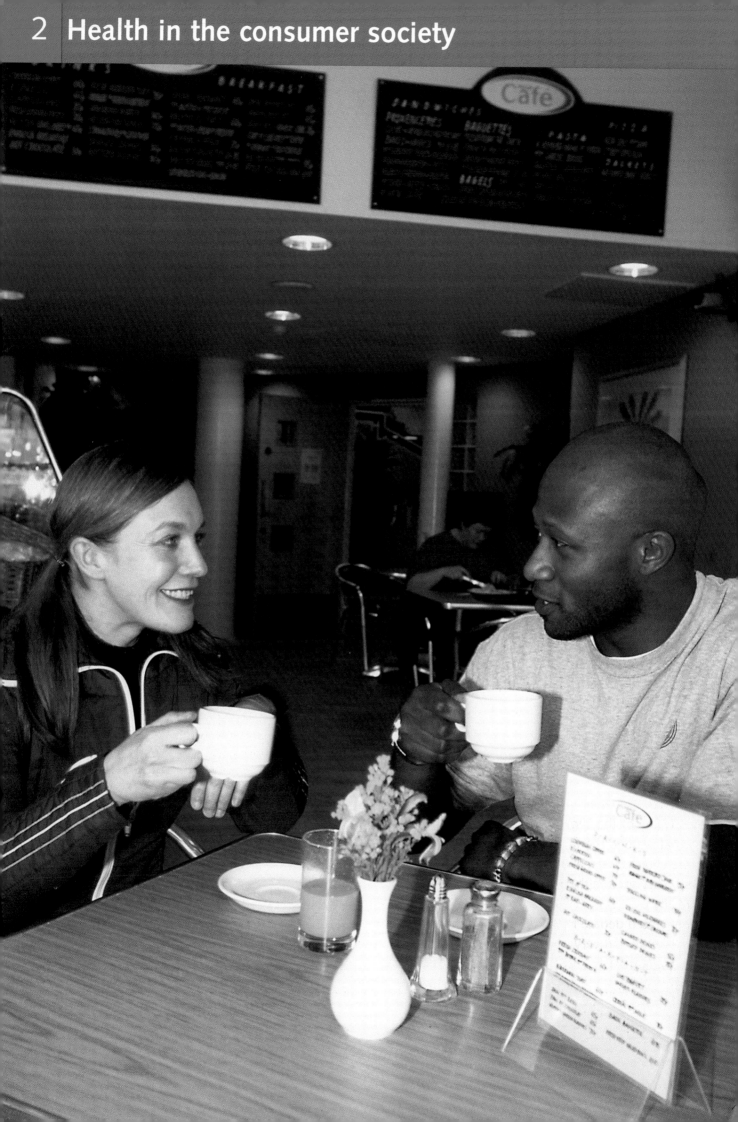

CHAPTER SUMMARY

- *The choices people make as consumers – what we eat and drink, and how we use services and facilities – impact on health.*

- *People get information on health from many different sources including friends and family, product labelling, the media, and national campaigns. A modern strategy for health will include action to stimulate both demand for healthier options – through information that people trust – as well as increase availability of those options, so that people can make the choices they want to.*

- *Action to address inequalities in health needs to focus particularly on getting information across to people in different groups and securing better access to healthier choices for people in disadvantaged groups or areas.*

- *Where demand for healthier choices is increasing – for example following the national campaigns on 5 A DAY and on salt – industry is already responding.*

- *The Government has a role in taking the lead on issues where strong national and public concern about health indicates the need to do more. This includes coordinated action with industry to increase awareness of the benefits and supply of healthy options – in particular supporting opportunities for exercise and a healthy diet – and action to reduce demand for less healthy foods, tobacco and alcohol, particularly among children and young people.*

INTRODUCTION

1. Many of the choices that affect our health – what we eat, the facilities and services we use – are choices we make as consumers. A modern strategy for health needs to deal directly with this reality of everyone's lives. The consultation generated debate between producers, retailers, the marketing industry, the media, communities and individuals about how to make choosing health an easier option.

2. Consumers play a major role in developing choices within the market. But there are other factors involved in developing the market opportunities on offer for health. To maximise the number of people making healthy choices, both consumer demand and market provision need to be influenced.

3. People want information about what they can do that will make a difference to their health, as well as access to the options that can help them in

adopting a healthy lifestyle – choice in what they eat, how and where they take exercise, and in how they access support services. Government has a role in fostering demand for health, working with public services, the voluntary sector and industry to get accurate information and choices to people in ways that are relevant to their lives and meet their needs as individuals.

4. Differences of income and wealth mean that market systems – which are designed to promote choice – bring inequalities in terms of opportunities to make healthy choices in where we live, what food we eat and how we spend our leisure time. Deprived communities often lack good local access to places to buy fresh fruit and vegetables, safe parks and playgrounds for exercise, or a full range of local health improvement services. People living in temporary accommodation may lack adequate facilities to prepare healthy meals.

5. Systems which work well for most people, whatever their income, bring other sorts of inequality. Poor presentation of information on food labels can mean that people are not aware of which foods are high in constituents such as fat that are harmful if eaten to excess. Some people have difficulty in using the information that is available because they suffer from learning or physical disabilities, lack basic literacy skills, or cannot read English.

6. Wider cross-government action, including action on employment and tackling social exclusion, plays its part in equalising opportunities and reducing inequalities. There is also a growing interest in how society can seek to influence the market in the interests of health.

7. People believe that in a market economy it is not a matter for Government to dictate to them what they can and cannot consume. But they recognise that there may be exceptions on grounds of safety or where the choices people make can have significant consequences for others, and that there is a special case for protecting children.

CREATING A DEMAND FOR HEALTHY CHOICES

8. A wide range of lifestyle choices are marketed to people, but health itself has not been marketed. Promoting health on the principles that commercial markets use – making it something people aspire to and making healthy choices enjoyable and convenient – will create a stronger demand for health and in turn influence industry to take more account of broader health issues in what they produce.

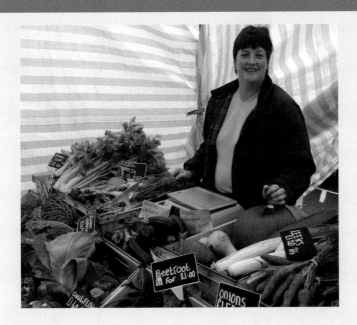

'...there was acknowledgement that the public could become confused with conflicting advice, particularly in relation to things that are declared good for you, and then bad, by turns.'

King's Fund

Marketing health

9. We need to learn much more about how to both create and respond to demand for health nationally and within local communities. Alcohol and fast food are portrayed as offering excitement, escape and instant gratification. Television, computer games and the sofa offer attractive entertainment options. In contrast, the portrayal of healthy lifestyles by government can seem preachy, boring and too much like hard work.

10. The *Choosing Health?* consultation took evidence from people who help make the less healthy choices the sexy ones – marketers and advertisers. They told us that the power of 'social marketing', marketing tools applied to social good, could be used to build public awareness and change behaviour, making behaviour that harms health less attractive and encouraging behaviour that builds health. To be effective in influencing demand for health, marketing messages need to be given, received, believed, understood and acted on.

Getting the message across to people

11. The problem is not lack of information on what is good for you and what is not – people are getting new 'facts' from all sides. But messages about health are sometimes inconsistent or uncoordinated and out of step with the way people actually live their lives.

12. Once we have a clear message about health, it is important that people can act on it. National and local government, the voluntary and community sectors and industry are beginning to develop new partnerships: to communicate more consistent messages on health and ensure that people can follow them up easily. This approach proved successful in the 5 A DAY programme. The Department of Health took the lead in establishing clear and consistent criteria on what food counts towards 5 A DAY based on scientific evidence. But we relied on partners in industry to get messages across to consumers and to respond to consumer needs by making fruit and vegetables available in convenient formats and locations. We intend now to simplify messages on what a portion means for children and adults, for example, using 'a handful'.

5 A DAY communication programme

- The programme provides information and advice for consumers through a wide range of routes – television and radio 'filler' advertising, printed resources including leaflets, posters, booklets, a website, PR and magazine adverts and articles.
- 5 A DAY is promoted in the NHS, where the radio fillers are being played widely across hospital radio stations, and with communications activity targeting hospital caterers.
- The 5 A DAY logo is the first government-licensed logo, supported by clear criteria on how it can be used. It is used by over 400 organisations and on many products with high volume sales.
- Consumer research commissioned by the Department of Health, Department for Environment, Food and Rural Affairs (DEFRA) and Food Standards Agency (FSA) indicates:
  - People trust messages they get from retailers in a way that they don't trust government.
  - A year-on-year increase in awareness of the 5 A DAY message from 52% in October 2002 to 59% in October 2003.
  - Consumption of fresh fruit rose by 5.8% between 2001–02 and 2002–03.

13. The Department of Health will lead on action to promote health by influencing people's attitudes to the choices they make through a strategy that extends across all aspects of health and involves a broad range of different government departments and agencies such as those covering interests in the NHS, food, sport, the environment and transport. The Department of Health will appoint an independent body to implement the strategy on its behalf.

14. The strategy will include new communications which build on previous successful campaigns on smoking, salt, mental wellbeing and sexual health, and extend to include information on obesity, healthy eating and physical activity in different groups.

15. We will bring together messages that raise awareness of health risks with information about action that people can take themselves to address those risks – for example, by changing their diet, taking more exercise or seeking advice through telephone helplines, local health improvement services. Early focus will be on:

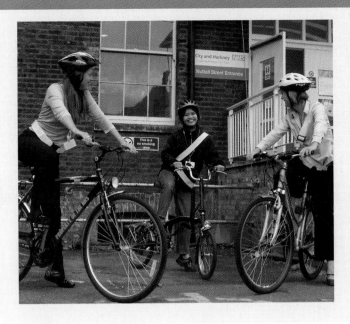

- *sexual health* – with a new national campaign targeted particularly at younger men and women to ensure that they understand the real risk of unprotected sex, and persuade them of the benefits of using condoms to avoid the risk of sexually transmitted infections (STIs) or unplanned pregnancies;
- *obesity* – a new cross-government campaign to raise awareness of the health risks of obesity, and the steps people can take through diet and physical activity to prevent obesity;
- *smoking* – a boosted campaign to reduce smoking rates and motivate smokers in different groups to quit supported by clear and comprehensive information about health risks, reasons not to smoke, and access to NHS support to quit, including Stop Smoking Services and nicotine replacement therapy;
- *alcohol* – working with the Portman Group[1] to cut down binge drinking.

These campaigns will operate at a national and regional level and use creative social marketing techniques and new technology. They will promote key messages and local services through a variety of channels, for example in schools and workplaces as well as through health professionals.

16. In the longer term we expect to see a significant part of the strategy delivered through campaigns that are jointly funded by government and industry.

17. Any strategy for promoting health – whether through campaigns or changes in service provision – must be based on an understanding of what different population groups need. This means taking account of why people make the choices they do – for example, information on diet and nutrition or dealing with stress needs to be tailored differently to first time parents, African-Caribbean men, older people in deprived communities, those from different socio-economic groups or people whose first language is not English. They will also need to be effective in tackling addictive behaviour, such as smoking. Each element of any new campaign will be based on the best available evidence and international best practice and tested to ensure that the messages get across to the relevant target audience.

BETTER INFORMATION TO SUPPORT HEALTHY CHOICES IN A CONSUMER SOCIETY

18. Success in developing demand for health is not enough on its own; people need to be able to make informed choices about what action to take.

Clear information that people trust

19. Information about health will always be available from a range of different sources. The Government's role is to help information providers

1   The Portman Group was set up in 1989 by the UK's leading drinks producers to promote responsible drinking, help prevent misuse of alcohol, encourage responsible marketing, and foster a balanced understanding of alcohol-related issues.

CASE STUDY

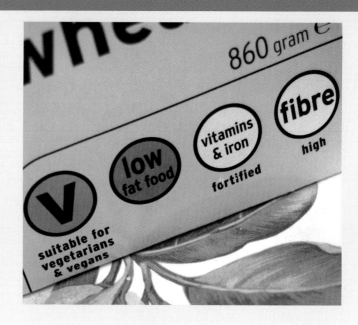

Action Diabetes is a programme run by Slough Primary Care Trust, working with Dr Foster, the health information specialists. It uses an approach which combines data on hospital admissions with demographic data by area down to neighbourhood level, to identify which communities generate most admissions consistent with late diagnosis of Type 2 diabetes. This information is used to devise ways to communicate with those patients who are most at risk of health complications and acute episodes which require emergency treatment.

The pilot identified a largely Asian community, living in economically stressed circumstances and often without English, which shopped locally at discount retailers and had a high propensity to watch the local cable television shopping channel. So to raise awareness of diabetes, building a relationship with local discount retailers and communicating via cable television makes good marketing sense. An Action Diabetes bus is already taking testing and health promotion services out to schools, temples, mosques, businesses and community centres. There are also videos and magazines now being produced and trained voluntary health counsellors will work within local communities to provide advice to those most at risk on how to obtain information on diabetes and improving health.

give factual information that is up to date and accurate.

20. The Department of Health is already working with providers of information on healthcare to:

- add the NHS brand and other brands, such as 5 A DAY, to high-quality health information resources; and
- help distribute them – for example, working with the Coalition for Cancer and through other campaigns.

21. The most successful campaigns have been those that reach people through a number of sources that actively and consistently promote health. We will build on this by:

- **funding specific campaigns through non-governmental organisations like the British Heart Foundation, Cancer Research UK and Age Concern;**
- **encouraging industry involvement – through use of consistent messages on health like 5 A DAY in supermarkets and on food packaging – to reach people when they are making choices;**
- **working with the sports and recreational activity sectors to deliver positive, innovative messages about healthy lifestyles through, for example, football, walking, cycling and fitness centres;**

'Food labelling is a tool that could potentially enable consumers to choose healthier foods and negotiate their way through today's "obesogenic society" more successfully. However, current labelling appears to fall far short of this aim.'

Health Select Committee Report on Obesity

■ linking into activity in communities, schools and workplaces to make messages relevant to different people's lives – as set out in chapters 3, 4 and 6.

Information on food content

22. Food is a prime example of an area where there needs to be clear and consistent information to help people make healthy choices. A lot of information is provided on packaged and processed foods. Many people already understand the importance of thinking about how much salt, fat and sugar they eat. But lists expressed in terms that few of us can understand are not enough. What we need to know is where a particular food fits in a healthy balanced diet so that we can make informed choices.

23. **We will press vigorously for progress before and during the UK presidency of the EU in 2005 to simplify nutrition labelling and make it mandatory on packaged foods.**

Nutritional criteria

24. The Department of Health has started work with the FSA to develop criteria that take account of fat, salt and sugar levels to indicate the contribution a food makes to a healthy balanced diet. **By mid-2005 we aim to have introduced a system that could be used as a standard basis for signposting foods. This will build on the nutrient**

criteria for the 5 A DAY logo. The criteria will also be used among other things to identify which foods can be promoted to children (see paragraphs 48–52). The criteria for use of the 5 A DAY logo will be extended to processed foods and to foods targeted at children.

Signposting food

25. Some retailers are already considering different signposting approaches for food on the front of packaging in response to consumer demand. The aim of signposting foods is to make it easier for people to see at a glance how individual foods contribute to a healthy balanced diet. The form of signposting can vary.

26. **The Government will work with the food industry to develop the signposting approach further on the completion of FSA consumer research. Our goal is, by early 2006, for there to be:**

■ **a clear, straightforward coding system**
■ **that is in common use, and**
■ **that busy people can understand at a glance which foods can make a positive contribution to a healthy diet, and which are recommended to be eaten only in moderation or sparingly.**

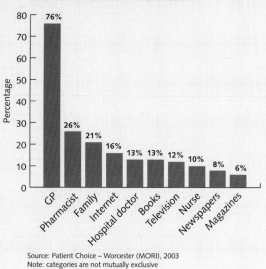

Sources of health information

Source: Patient Choice – Worcester (MORI), 2003
Note: categories are not mutually exclusive

Improved pack warnings for tobacco products

27. The stark warnings on tobacco products that we introduced in 2003 have had a real impact, but over time people become used to them. Evidence from countries that have picture warnings is that they are a powerful way of communicating the risks of smoking. **We believe that picture warnings on tobacco products could play a powerful role in any campaign to reduce the number of smokers and we will consult on how to use them most effectively when the European Commission publishes its final proposals.**

Information that is readily accessible

28. People get information about health from a wide range of sources beyond the doctor's surgery – friends and families, stories in newspapers and magazines or on television, the internet, voluntary sector organisations, public advice centres and libraries, schools, sports centres and shops. For example, news pages and lifestyle sections of newspapers, magazines and the broadcast media, regularly cover topics such as obesity, diet, exercise and smoking.

29. NHS Direct, fully established in 2000, already provides general help and advice to some 7 million people each year through a telephone helpline and through 6.5 million visits to the NHS Direct Online website. The most recent developments include

extending NHS Direct services through digital television channels, information on local services through www.nhs.uk and including health information in Thomson Local directories.

30. We will commission a new service – Health Direct – to provide easily accessible and confidential information on health choices. Health Direct will be set up from 2007. It will include links to existing services, for example information on diet and nutrition (provided by the FSA) and support for parents (provided by Sure Start and other agencies).

31. Health Direct will be developed as a telephone, internet and digital television service. It will also be available to people who do not have internet access at home through the Government-funded UK Online centres. These centres provide internet access, at zero or low cost, in a range of convenient community venues where users can get support to access government services online.

Information on health in the media

32. Newspapers, television and radio were active protagonists in the *Choosing Health?* consultation and extended its reach both nationally and locally. Many broadcasters – including ITV and the BBC – have run programming strands and campaigns designed to get people thinking about their health. As part of *Choosing Health?*, the Department of

CASE STUDY

What Now? provides information and advice services to young people as part of Lancashire County Council's Youth and Community Service. This includes the provision of interactive services for young people that offer advice on everything from the impact of drug taking to bullying and getting a better education. A freephone helpline, webchat, e-mail and text enquiry service is available every day of the year, from 10am to 10pm, providing information, advice and support to young people on 'anything that concerns them'.

Staff are all qualified youth and community workers who specialise in information and advice work. Thanks to its flexibility, giving teenagers support when they need it most, the service has been purchased on a subscription basis by a number of other local authorities and the DfES Connexions partnerships across England.

Health commissioned the King's Fund to undertake a brief consultation directly with the media, to test how they saw their role and whether there were approaches that might encourage continued and responsible coverage of health issues.

From the national media there were clear views on its distinctive role:

"The task of the media is to hold the ring as much as it can sorting out the competing demands of the various players – individuals, professions and government – and enable the debate to determine the acceptable level of government intervention."
Deputy editor, Sunday broadsheet

33. Among the regional media, there was much greater willingness to engage in coverage to promote information and debate about particular issues. Their responsibility to their local readers was more likely to see them engaged as active participants in the drive to improve standards of health:

"It is one of the biggest issues facing our country and the people in this area – there's a lot of eating pies and chips, drinking and smoking tabs here, and it's got to be tackled."
Editor, regional evening paper, North East England

"There's nothing more satisfying. I'm sure we've saved lives of people in our area and improved

health. I think we are very proud of that."
Editor, regional morning paper, North Yorkshire and North East England

34. The scale of media interest in topics such as obesity, diet, exercise and smoking is plain and there is an appetite for more accurate and accessible information. The Government will of course continue to provide information on health-related issues through departmental press offices and new resources such as Health Direct. **From the beginning of 2005, the Department of Health will:**

- **expand the existing programme of expert briefings provided by the Chief Medical Officer to include regular and coordinated updates on a wider range of health-related topics; and**
- **provide support for the development of an independent regular forum with regional and national media to discuss major health issues – a national centre for media and health.**

Redressing inequalities in access to information to tackle disadvantage

35. We also need to look at ways to make healthy choices more accessible to individuals and groups who may not find it easy to use information designed to meet the needs of the general population. **We will look to providers of local services to:**

- take account of the factors that impact on the decisions people make about their health;
- tailor information and advice to meet people's needs and support staff to communicate complex health information to different groups in the population;
- provide practical support for people who lack basic skills to help them use health information, including signposting them to extra support; and
- build new opportunities for health – such as the electronic patient record and *HealthSpace* – into education and development provided in further education and in the workplace.

> - A survey of readability of patient information produced by hospices and palliative care units in the UK showed that 64% of leaflets were readable only by an estimated 40% of the population.

Working with individuals to improve understanding of health

> **2003 national research study for the DfES**
> - 5.2 million adults in England could be described as lacking basic literacy (that is, they were at entry level 3 or below according to National Standards for Literacy and Numeracy).
> - More than one-third of people with poor or very poor health had literacy skills of entry level 3 or below.
> - Low levels of literacy and numeracy were found to be associated with socio-economic deprivation.
> - 53% of all adults surveyed had entry or lower level practical skills in using information and communication technology (ICT).

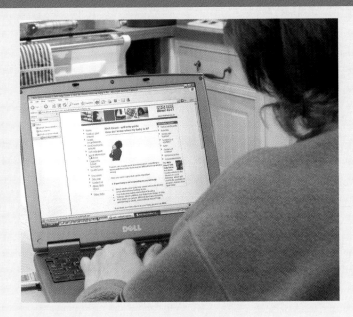

The Prime Minister launched *Skills for Life* – the national strategy for improving adult literacy, language (English for Speakers of Other Languages) and numeracy skills – in March 2001. The strategy sets out how the Government plans to tackle the problem of people with poor basic skills. The goal is to improve the skills of 2.25 million adults by 2010, with interim targets of 750,000 by 2004 and 1.5 million by 2007.

36. We are taking action to help people develop their understanding of health issues. *Skilled for Health*[2] combines the national adult basic skills programme, *Skills for Life*,[3] with tackling people's needs for a better understanding of their health. The programme provides practical help in managing situations, such as making an appointment with a doctor, or calculating a dosage of medicine. It is helping parents improve their reading skills while they help their own children to learn.

37. **To drive forward action to improve people's understanding of health issues, focusing first on the most deprived areas, we will:**

- **provide new funding to enable every NHS primary care trust by 2007 to run at least one local *Skilled for Health* programme each year as part of local strategies for health;**
- **expand *Skilled for Health*, with a further wave of projects in workplaces in partnership with Business in the Community, focusing on marginalised groups where people commonly lack basic skills;**
- **introduce courses on what the new electronic patient care record does and how to use it in planning personal health choices.[4] These courses will be included in relevant learning curricula for adult education;**
- **expand access to training, advice and education to support individuals to develop skills in improving their own health; and**
- **draw on the specialist skills of relevant organisations to develop action on health literacy.[5]**

---

2   *Skilled for Health* is a partnership between DH, DfES and the learning charity ContinYou.

3   DfES: *Skills for Life: the national strategy for improving adult literacy and numeracy skills*, 2000, www.dfes.gov.uk/readwriteplus/

4   The roll-out of a nationally accessible electronic patient care record started in autumn 2004. The pace of roll-out will accelerate throughout 2005.

5   Led by the Department of Health this could include among others: the National Consumer Council, ContinYou, the National Institute of Adult Continuing Education (NIACE), the National Institute for Clinical Excellence (NICE), NHSU, the Learning and Skills Council and the Institute of Education.

CASE STUDY

A *Skilled for Health* project, jointly funded by Thurrock Primary Care NHS Trust and Thurrock Adult Community College (Essex), provides outreach support to less advantaged parents with young children who have literacy and numeracy needs. The project is part of a well-established and innovative Community Mothers parent support programme and enables parents with young children to access learning provision or one-to-one basic skills support in their own homes. New health and parenting skills are gained as an integral part of the basic skills tuition.

A mother who took part in the project said, "When I looked at healthy eating it showed me what I was eating was not that healthy, I was having more fats than I should and I did not realise a portion size was so much. I would have not known where to go for information about this. My family are now having a healthier diet. When I go shopping I know what to look for on labels."

DEMAND FOR HEALTH AS AN INFLUENCE IN THE MARKET

Consumer influence and corporate social responsibility

38. The first part of this chapter has focused on creating demand for health through marketing campaigns, and making it easier for individuals to choose healthy lifestyles in a consumer society. Individuals and communities can also influence markets through the health choices they make.

39. For markets to work many thousands of people have to want a product. If consumers act together as a group, they can have a great deal of power. The consultation highlighted abundant evidence that groups of consumers can do a lot to influence others, and that industry and the market respond to such influences.

40. The public expects big organisations to be socially responsible corporate citizens, an expectation that industry is increasingly recognising. Many corporate organisations acknowledge that what they do for the community impacts on their reputation and that meeting these expectations can make good business sense. We recognise, for example, the commitment that retailers and food producers have already made towards promoting healthier eating and the scope that exists within the food industry's policies and

'Corporate social responsibility (CSR) can be a powerful tool for good when it is driven by values, and is applied meaningfully and consistently across a company's activities. There is clearly scope for the exercise of CSR to be strengthened by the independent development of standards and independent monitoring and scrutiny, and there is a role for governments at national and international levels to play in this process. It is society that has to pick up the extrinsic costs of commercial activities.'

National Heart Forum

practices for further activity to 'eat well, drink well'. **This includes action in four key areas:**

- **Product development** – assessing market opportunities and making sure that the development of healthier foods, including 'own brand' products, meet customer requirements for affordability, convenience and taste, for example, in salt, fat and sugar content of foods.
- **Labelling information** – by developing nutrition labelling and associated messages such as 5 A DAY, well beyond legal requirements, some retailers are already helping customers make informed choices.
- **Promotion and pricing** – communication strategies to promote healthier eating, including fruit and vegetables, through point of sale information, leaflets and websites.
- **Customer information and advice** – including healthy eating and the promotion of sensible drinking messages to combat alcohol misuse.

41. Recognising that the public sector can never provide all the answers, we have been encouraged by industry's commitment to working with us to improve the nutritional quality of food. But such commitments must deliver real change.

DRIVING FORWARD CHANGE
Developing partnerships with industry to promote health

42. In many areas consumer demand and better information, supported by strategies to market health, will be sufficient to secure the changes needed to improve health. But where urgent action is needed to tackle issues that are of national public concern – such as obesity or the increase in prevalence of diabetes and heart disease – the effect of market forces and corporate social responsibility are not enough on their own. Government has a role in engaging in the debate to speed up the natural pace of change.

43. **The Government intends to discuss with the food industry how they might contribute to funding national campaigns and other national initiatives to promote positive health information and education.**

44. **Health ministers and the FSA are leading discussions with industry to identify and implement a range of proposals to increase opportunities for people to make healthy choices in what they eat. These are aimed at:**

CASE STUDY

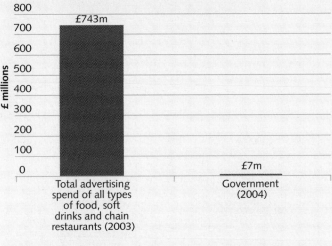

Advertising spend on food by industry compared to food campaign spend by Government

£743m

£7m

Total advertising spend of all types of food, soft drinks and chain restaurants (2003)

Government (2004)

Source on industry spend: Ofcom

The Food and Drink Federation's recently published *Food and Health Manifesto* sets out agreed members' commitments across seven key areas where food manufacturers, working with the rest of the food chain and other partners, will coordinate their efforts. The manifesto includes a commitment to 'continuing to reduce levels of sugar, fat and salt in products'.

Under Project Neptune, which is an industry-wide sodium reduction programme in the soups and sauces sector, encouraging progress has already been made. For example, the Association of Cereal Food Manufacturers, which has already reduced the salt in breakfast cereals by 22% between 1998 and 2003, intends to make further commitments to reductions in 2005.

- **increasing the availability of healthier food, including reducing the levels of salt, added sugars and fat in prepared and processed food and drink and increasing access to fruit and vegetables;**
- **reversing the trend towards bigger portion sizes; and**
- **adopting consistent and clear standards for information on food including signposting.**

45. **We will work with industry to develop voluntary action based on:**

- **long-term and interim targets for reducing sugar and fat levels in different categories of foods[6] – compliance will be monitored through regular surveys; and**
- **development of guidance on portion sizes to reduce energy, fat, sugar and salt intake.**

46. As a society we need to see significant change if we are going to be successful in tackling the health challenges set out in Chapter 1. **We will work with the farming and food industries to coordinate action, including action to take forward policies in this White Paper, through a *Food and Health Action Plan* to be published in early 2005 fulfilling the commitment to such a plan in our *Strategy for Sustainable Farming and Food*.[7] This will be backed up with wider action in the *Food Standards Agency Strategic Plan*.[8]**

6   This will build on the current FSA modelling framework developed for salt reduction.
7   Published December 2002, available at: www.defra.gov.uk/farm/sustain/default.htm
8   www.food.gov.uk/foodindustry/Consultations/completed_consultations/compconsulteng/promofoodconsult

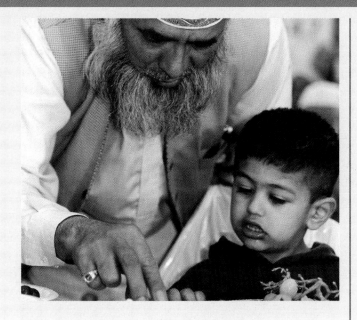

CASE STUDY

Protecting children and young people

47. Responses to the *Choosing Health?* consultation indicated that whilst people felt it was generally right to leave lifestyle choices up to each individual, the government should take specific steps to protect children and help them to make healthier choices. Even those commentators who felt it was inappropriate for the Government to take a role in encouraging adults to make more healthy choices felt it was appropriate to intervene with children.

Food promotion

48. When it comes to food, people feel that it is wrong for children to be bombarded with sophisticated marketing that might confuse them and reduces their ability to make healthy choices before they have been able to develop the skills and experience to negotiate their way through the array of choices on offer. In the responses to *Choosing Health?* there was overwhelming support for some restrictions on the marketing of unhealthy food and drinks to children.

49. The FSA commissioned a *Review of Research on the Effects of Food Promotion to Children*.[9] This review found that children's food promotion is dominated by television advertising, and that most of the research has focused on this area. However, it found that this research may 'understate the

Sid the slug is a sympathetic character created to front the public health campaign launched by the FSA in September 2004. The aim of the campaign is to save lives, by reducing the amount of salt people eat in the UK. Sid has appeared in all television, national poster and print advertising and on the dedicated campaign website: www.salt.gov.uk. Too much salt can raise your blood pressure, which increases your chances of developing heart disease and stroke. Every year there are 170,000 deaths in England alone where high blood pressure is a cause or contributing factor.

FSA Chairman Sir John Krebs said, "Many in the food industry have introduced salt reduction programmes and, to their credit, many major retailers and manufacturers now label products with the salt content.

"The food industry is about two-thirds of the way to reaching our target of a 1g reduction in processed foods by the end of 2005. However, to reach the ambitious target of 6g per day by 2010 will require further action by both consumers and industry if we are to reduce the human and health costs of eating too much salt."

---

9   *Review of Research on the Effects of Food Promotion to Children*, published September 2003, available at: www.food.gov.uk/multimedia/pdfs/foodpromotiontochildren1.pdf

"Please think about limiting junk food advertising on TV which is targeted at children. Adults make their own choices about their health, children are vulnerable and it's all too easy for adults to give in. My kids say 'I want, I want' when adverts are on the TV."

Mother

"I think that young people do understand that obesity and excessive weight gain is harmful to health but they find it difficult to maintain a healthy diet as they are constantly surrounded by junk food."

Young person

effect that food promotion has on children' and 'the cumulative effect of television advertising combined with other forms of promotion and marketing is likely to be significantly greater' than television alone. It concluded that 'food promotion can have and is having an effect on children, particularly in the areas of food preferences, purchase behaviour and consumption' and that 'these effects are significant, independent of other influences and operate at both a brand and category level'.

50. The Office of Communications (Ofcom), which regulates broadcasting and already has some restrictions on food promotion to children commissioned research[10] into its impact. Their report focused on the effects of television advertising of products high in fat, salt and sugar (HFSS) to children.

Ofcom concluded that television has *'modest direct effects on children's food choices. While indirect effects are likely to be larger, there is insufficient evidence to determine the relative size of the effect of TV advertising on children's food choices by comparison with other relevant factors.'*

51. On the basis of their research, Ofcom's overall conclusion is that there is a need for some specific and targeted tightening of the rules on television advertising, in the context of other changes.

However, Ofcom also concluded that a total ban on television advertising of food and drinks to children would be neither proportionate nor, in isolation, effective.

In addition, the report made a number of observations in relation to children's viewing patterns and found that:

- an average child watches around 17 hours of television each week (including non-commercial broadcasting);
- younger children see more advertising for core category products (ie foods, soft drinks, chain restaurants) in children's airtime than older children (eg 4–9 year olds see just over half of the core category adverts that they are exposed to during children's airtime); and
- children spend 71% of their viewing time outside children's airtime, with more children and young people watching television at peak times (between 6pm–9pm) than at any other part of the day.

In the *Choosing Health?* consultation, although some respondents called for an outright ban, some discussed restrictions during peak times for children's viewing.

52. But we need to look at all food advertising and promotion that is aimed at children. **In line with the research conclusions and the responses to the**

10 www.ofcom.org.uk/research/consumer_audience_research/tv/food_ads/

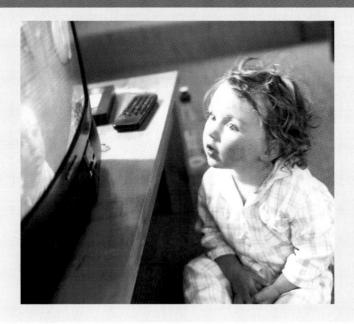

consultation, the Government considers there is a strong case for action to restrict further the advertising and promotion to children of those foods and drinks that are high in fat, salt and sugar. To have maximum effect, action needs to be comprehensive and taken in relation to all forms of food advertising and promotion, including:

- broadcast;
- non-broadcast;
- sponsorship and brand-sharing;[11]
- point of sale advertising, including vending in schools; and
- labels, wrappers and packaging.

53. Most of current advertising spend is through television. In 2003 advertisers for food, soft drinks and chain restaurants spent 72% of their budget promoting their products on television, making this a key medium for food advertisers.

54. There is a range of ways in which the rules governing food and drink advertising and promotion could be enhanced and strengthened. These might cover:

- when, where and how frequently certain advertisements and promotions appear – for example, an option would be to consider different restrictions during children's television (pre 6pm), during peak times (6pm–9pm) and after the 9pm watershed;

- the use of cartoon characters, role models, celebrities and glamorisation of foods that children should only eat seldom or in moderation as part of a balanced diet; and
- the inclusion of clear nutritional information – perhaps based on a signposting system – and/or balancing messages in advertisements to counteract the influence of high fat, salt and sugar food advertisements.

Options will be dependent upon the nutrient profiling scheme being developed by the Department of Health and the Food Standards Agency discussed earlier in this chapter.

Ofcom's recent tightening of rules governing alcohol advertising is a good example of regulation evolving and modernising to keep up with changes in society and marketing techniques.

55. The Government is keen to see real progress in this area. **On television, we will work with the broadcasting and advertising sectors on ways to help drive down levels of childhood obesity. In particular we will look to Ofcom to consult on proposals on tightening the rules on broadcast advertising, sponsorship and promotion of food and drink and securing their effective implementation by broadcasters in order to ensure that children are properly protected from encouragement to eat too many high fat, salt and**

11 Brand-sharing is the use of non-food products to promote a food product and vice versa.

"We believe that working to reduce alcohol misuse is in the interests of the drinks industry as well as of consumers and society in general. The leading companies who support our work understand that social responsibility is a key part of successful business strategies in today's society.

We have a strong shared agenda with government in promoting responsible drinking and responsible marketing practices. The Portman Group is therefore fully committed to working with government and the public health community towards our common objectives, particularly tackling binge drinking among young people."

Jean Coussins, Chief Executive, The Portman Group

sugar foods – both during children's programmes and at other times when large numbers of children are watching. It should also include options for broadcasters and advertisers to participate in healthy living promotions.

56. Marketing spend is not limited to television advertising and, indeed, may be increasing in other areas: this increase would probably be magnified when broadcast restrictions are increased unless a more comprehensive approach is adopted. Government is therefore also keen to see stronger controls on non-broadcast and other types of marketing. **We will work with industry, advertisers, consumer groups and other stakeholders to encourage new measures to strengthen existing voluntary codes in non-broadcast areas, including:**

- **setting up a new food and drink advertising and promotion forum to review, supplement, strengthen and bring together existing provisions; and**
- **contributing funding to the development of new health initiatives, including positive health campaigns.**

57. There was a clear call in the responses to *Choosing Health?* for restrictions on the promotion and sponsorship of food and drink in schools. As noted in the *Healthy Living Blueprint*[12] launched

earlier this year, a challenge for schools is to balance the benefits of food promotional activity – including sponsorship, advertising and branding of materials – with the ethos of a healthy school and whole school approach to healthy eating. This will be considered further as part of the comprehensive approach outlined above.

58. **The Government is committed to ensuring that measures to protect children's health are rigorously implemented and soundly based on evidence of impact. We will therefore monitor the success of these measures in relation to the balance of food and drink advertising and promotion to children, and children's food preferences to assess their impact. If, by early 2007, they have failed to produce change in the nature and balance of food promotion, we will take action through existing powers or new legislation to implement a clearly defined framework for regulating the promotion of food to children.**

59. In addition, there are a range of creative ways for positive campaigns to promote healthy lifestyles in order to counteract the impact of advertising of high fat, sugar and salt foods, and Government is keen to see these used by industry. We will look to the broadcasting and advertising sectors, including Ofcom, to consider how they could have a positive impact on children's food choices. The power of

12 www.teachernet.gov.uk/healthyliving/

broadcasting could be harnessed, such as in recent campaigns like ITV's *Britain on the Move*. Marketing devices such as cartoon characters, role models, celebrities and glamorisation could also be used to promote foods that children should eat more often.

Alcohol and health

60. The Portman Group[13] has already created a mechanism to use some of the profits of the alcohol industry's success in the market place to promote health messages. **We will work in partnership with the Portman Group to develop a new and strengthened information campaign to tackle the problems of binge drinking.**

61. **We will also work with industry to develop a voluntary social responsibility scheme for alcohol producers and retailers to protect young people by:**

- **placing information for the public on alcohol containers and in alcohol retail outlets;**
- **including reminders about responsible drinking on alcohol advertisements; and**
- **checking identification and refusing to sell alcohol to people who are under 18.**

62. During the development of the *Alcohol Harm Reduction Strategy for England*, concerns were raised about the effectiveness of the current rules on alcohol advertising, which are aimed mainly at preventing an inappropriate influence on children and people under 18 and at preventing advertising condoning anti-social or self-destructive behaviour by any age group. **Ofcom, which has statutory responsibility for the regulation of broadcast advertising, has been undertaking a review of the rules on broadcast advertising of alcohol and has published its code amendments, aimed at significantly strengthening the rules in many areas, particularly to protect the under-18s.**

63. The new rules, which will take effect from 1 January 2005, include requirements that:

- advertisements for alcoholic drinks on television must not be likely to appeal strongly to people under 18, in particular by reflecting or being associated with youth culture;
- advertisements must not link alcohol with sexual activity or success or imply that alcohol can enhance attractiveness;
- television advertising for alcoholic drinks must not show, imply, or refer to daring, toughness, aggression or unruly, irresponsible or anti-social behaviour; and
- alcoholic drinks must be handled and served responsibly in television advertising.

13 www.portman-group.org.uk/alcohol/47.asp.

CASE STUDY

Every year Quit runs a National Smoke-Free Ramadan Campaign with partners like the British Heart Foundation, Smoke-Free London, the Muslim Health Network and the imams of some 60 large mosques. The campaign reaches some 1.6 million Muslims in the UK. Last year's campaign was targeted at smokers and non-smokers alike during the Muslim holy month of fasting, to bring home the dangers of second-hand smoke to the family. Smokers were urged to stop smoking as they are twice as much at risk of developing heart diseases as non-smokers. Their family and colleagues were urged to support the smokers in their quit attempt as they too risk developing the same diseases as the smokers through second-hand smoke.

Tobacco advertising and promotion

64. In 2003 the Tobacco Advertising and Promotion Act put an end to almost all tobacco advertising, recognising the harmful nature of tobacco and the link between advertising and increased consumption.

- **By the end of the year the size of tobacco advertising still allowed in shops will be restricted to a total area the size of an A5 piece of paper – a third of which will be a health warning featuring the NHS Smoking Helpline number.**
- **In 2005 we will end internet advertising and brand-sharing (using a non-tobacco product) in the UK.**

65. The Government is aware of research that suggests that children and young people may be influenced to start smoking by viewing role models smoking in films, particularly if it is presented as a sophisticated, desirable activity. The British Board of Film Classification (BBFC) has assured the Government that it does consider whether a film targeted at children and young people is actively promoting smoking. The Board's classification guidelines are currently under consideration and one aspect of that review includes the public's attitude to smoking in films with particular appeal to children and young people, and the potential impact on their smoking behaviour.

66. We are pleased that there seems to have been a reduction in the portrayal of smoking on television in recent years. Broadcasters do appear to have followed the Independent Television Commission (now part of Ofcom) code rules; these require that smoking should be avoided in children's programmes and that, in other programmes likely to be widely seen by children and young people, smoking should be included only where context or dramatic veracity requires it, and even then not prominently featured as a normal or attractive activity. However, concerns have been put to us about the continued frequency of smoking in soap operas and its appearance in new formats such as reality programmes, often shown before the watershed. These programmes are popular with older children and young teenagers who may be influenced if role models are shown smoking or if it is shown in a positive light.

67. Ofcom has proposed a new broadcasting code which will come into effect in 2005. All broadcasters who are licensed by Ofcom, and the BBC and S4C, must comply with the relevant code. The proposed code contains rules about smoking in the section entitled 'protecting the under-18s', which clearly recognises the potential for harm and

the need for a clear framework for the way smoking is dealt with in programming where children are concerned. The Government welcomes Ofcom's consultation on this issue. In this consultation Ofcom has proposed tightening the rules so that smoking would be prohibited in children's programmes, unless there is a clear educational purpose, and in programmes before the watershed, unless there is an editorial justification. Ofcom is considering the wording of these rules and whether additional rules may be required in the light of responses and evidence they receive.

CONCLUSION

68. The actions in this chapter set out how we will work across government, with industry and other organisations to increase demand for health and support healthier choices with a comprehensive strategy to market health:

- providing people with clear information and advice about health choices in ways that can be easily understood and through channels that people use, as well as access to healthier choices;
- ensuring that the NHS and other public services develop responsive services where people want support or advice in adopting healthy lifestyles – targeting help and support to groups that are excluded, including those who need help in developing the basic skills to make healthy choices;
- influencing industry to promote healthier options and backing this up with a national *Food and Health Action Plan*; and
- protecting children and young people's health, in particular, through restrictions on market promotion of certain foods, alcohol and tobacco.

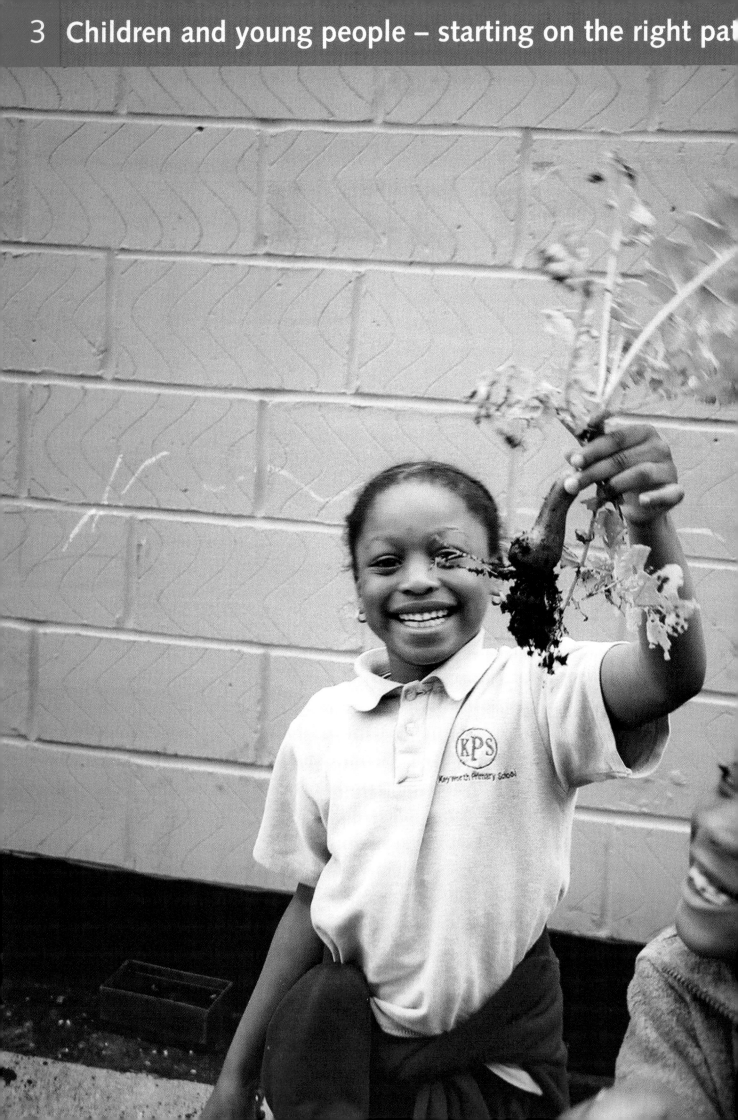

CHAPTER SUMMARY

This chapter sets out action to support children and young people, as well as their parents, families, carers and staff in the public and voluntary sectors. It aims to support development of a healthy framework for life.

- *There will be new sources of information guidance and practical support for parents, children and young people – particularly those who are disadvantaged in early years – provided in ways that are designed to meet their individual needs and be accessible to everyone.*
- *Services will be coordinated to meet needs and increasingly will be brought together in one location as part of an integrated service delivery through children's trust arrangements.*
- *The components of good health will be a core part of children's experience in schools through a coordinated 'whole school' approach to health – in lessons, sport, provision of food, personal advice and support, and travel arrangements.*
- *There will be new initiatives to promote physical activity and sport inside and outside school.*
- *We will strengthen measures to protect children and young people and help them understand and manage risk and develop responsible patterns of behaviour.*

INTRODUCTION

1. People's patterns of behaviour are often set early in life and influence their health throughout their lives. Infancy, childhood and young adulthood are critical stages in the development of habits that will affect people's health in later years.

2. This chapter outlines action to promote healthy choices early in life and to provide a supportive environment for children and young people themselves, as well as their parents, families and carers. It also sets out how the public and voluntary sectors can contribute. The actions aim to:

- reduce infant mortality;
- support all children and young people to attain good physical and mental health;
- reduce inequalities in opportunities for children to make healthy choices and address environmental inequalities that can undermine those choices; and
- ensure children and young people develop a good understanding of how they can balance the opportunities and risks in choices that impact on their health as they grow up.

'Increasingly, evidence is showing that children and young people do not play out as much as they used to and that their opportunities for free play are restricted.'

(Demos et al May 2004, Children's Play Council: Making the case for fair play, 2002)

3. We will integrate the action set out in this chapter with wider initiatives in the cross-government *Every Child Matters: Change for Children* programme,[1] which will involve local services, the voluntary and community sector, parents, carers and families. This approach will aim to improve the outcomes for all children – narrowing the gap between disadvantaged children and others.

Tackling deprivation and disadvantage in childhood

4. Most children now enjoy a healthy and positive start in life, but too many have poor physical or emotional health as a result of poverty and deprivation or poor parenting. This can result in lower life expectancy and poor mental health.

5. Our goal is to halve child poverty by 2010 and eradicate it by 2020. This will be achieved by a combination of hard work by people and the opportunities created by government. The Child Poverty Review[2] reinforced the importance of commitment across a wide range of public services to improving poor children's life chances and tackling cycles of deprivation. This includes initiatives that improve health outcomes for children, such as:

- delivering more decent homes;
- investment in early years services for disadvantaged children;
- increasing the take-up of sport and activity opportunities for children;
- reducing the proportion of women who smoke in pregnancy;
- extending the coverage of child and adolescent mental health services; and
- supporting parents.

6. Addressing health inequalities among children and young people has to be a major priority for all local agencies in order to break the cycle of deprivation that has undermined so many strategies for improving health in the past. **Subject to parliamentary approval, powers set out in the Children Bill will introduce the *Children and Young People's Plan*. The plan will bring together planning for local authority services with other plans, for example for health services, voluntary and community services and drugs action for children and young people.[3] We will look to primary care trusts (PCTs) to be fully involved with the new *Children and Young People's Plan* arrangements and to contribute advice and support in taking action to promote the health of children and young people.**

---

1   This programme will implement the reforms in the *Every Child Matters* Green Paper and the *National Service Framework for Children, Young People and Maternity Services* across government, local services, the voluntary and community sector, parents, carers and families. The aim of the programme is to deliver improved outcomes for all children and young people under the five headings of: be healthy; stay safe; enjoy and achieve; make a positive contribution; and achieve economic wellbeing.

2   www.hm-treasury.gov.uk/spending_review/spend_sr04/associated_documents/spending_sr04_childpoverty.cfm

3   Local authority directors of children's services will be responsible for drawing up *Children and Young People's Plans* locally.

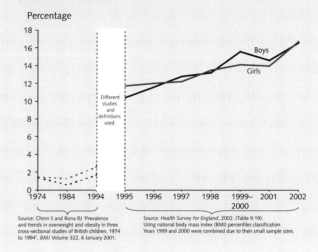

Obesity prevalence trends in children from 1974 to 2002 (from 1974 to 1994, primary school age; from 1995 to 2002, ages 2 to 15; England)

Percentage

Boys

Girls

Different studies and definitions used.

1974   1984   1994   1995   1996   1997   1998   1999–   2001   2002
                                                            2000

Source: Chinn S and Rona RJ 'Prevalence and trends in overweight and obesity in three cross-sectional studies of British children, 1974 to 1994', *BMJ* Volume 322, 6 January 2001.

Source: *Health Survey for England*, 2002. (Table 9.19). Using national body mass index (BMI) percentiles classification. Years 1999 and 2000 were combined due to their small sample sizes.

7. Looked-after children, disabled children and black and minority ethnic children often face more problems of health and wellbeing than others and are less likely to access services – such as immunisation programmes – that promote good health. The *National Service Framework for Children, Young People and Maternity Services* sets out the standards that local authorities and PCTs should follow in planning, commissioning and delivering services for children. The Summary of Intelligence on Inequalities discusses the action we are taking to tackle inequalities generally published with this White Paper.

Responding to changes in the way people live

8. Children need a balance of different opportunities in their lives to build the foundations of good physical and emotional health – opportunities that relate to the way people live in the 21st century.

9. Overall, many children appear to have fewer opportunities for physical activity and more are overweight – some obese. Some commentators suggest that this is because children are eating more convenience and fast foods, spending more time watching television or playing computer games, and less time being physically active because of the increase in car travel and a

heightened concern about the potential risks of unsupervised play outdoors.

> The prevalence of obesity in children aged 2 to 10 years has increased from 9.6% in 1995 to 15.5% in 2002 (*Health Survey for England* 2002). Obese children, especially girls, are more likely to come from lower social groups. Children who are obese are more likely to become obese adults, and this likelihood increases the more obese a child is, as well as increasing if the child's parents are obese.

10. Halting the growth in childhood obesity is our prime objective. **We have set a national target to halt, by 2010, the year-on-year increase in obesity among children under 11 in the context of a broader strategy to tackle obesity in the population as a whole. This objective will be shared jointly by the government departments with responsibility for health, education and sport.** Many of the initiatives in this White Paper will impact on obesity, including obesity in children – these are summarised in the Summary of Intelligence on Obesity published with this White Paper.

11. Modern technology, with information, entertainment and communication available at the touch of a button, increases opportunities to learn and explore ideas but can also diminish curiosity, initiative and enthusiasm for other things.

12. We need to offer children and young people more affordable, stimulating and accessible things to do outside the school day, at weekends and in school holidays that develop skills and extend healthy choices.

Building health in

13. Consultation made it clear that we need to create a culture where being concerned about health, including emotional wellbeing, asking for help or information and discussing risk is seen as natural behaviour that is respected and valued. This means responding better to what children, young people and their families want – developing the skills, knowledge, confidence and competence of everyone who works with them and providing a better coordinated approach to the health information and services on offer. It also means recognising that emotional wellbeing underpins good physical health and reduces the likelihood that children and young people will take inappropriate risks.

14. Following recommendations in *Every Child Matters*, the Department for Education and Skills (DfES) is developing a common core of skills and knowledge to support training for all professionals working with children, young people, families and carers. The common core will pay attention to the importance of promoting good health, and of recognising and being willing to discuss health concerns in response to requests.

DEVELOPING AN INTEGRATED FRAMEWORK FOR CHILD HEALTH

15. The first step towards developing a better response to children's health needs is the *Child Health Promotion* programme set out in the *National Service Framework for Children, Young People and Maternity Services*.[4] For the first time, this provides a joined-up system to ensure health and wellbeing for children and young people from birth to adulthood. The new programme moves on from a narrow focus on health screening and developmental reviews to a more broad-based programme of support to children and their families that will help address the wider determinants of health and reduce health inequalities. It puts in place a comprehensive system for health that focuses on priority issues such as diet and physical activity, safety, smoking and emotional wellbeing.[5] The programme covers:

- the assessment of the child's and family's needs;
- health promotion;

---

4   www.dh.gov.uk/PolicyAndGuidance/HealthAndSocialCareTopics/ChildrensServices/ChildServicesInformation/ChildrensServicesInformationArticle/fs/en?CONTENT_ID=4089111&chk=U8Ecln

5   National Service Framework (NSF) standards are developmental standards in the *Health and Social Care Standards and Planning Framework* and will therefore form part of the annual assessment undertaken by the Healthcare Commission. The standards in the NSF will need to be delivered in partnership with local authorities. Subject to parliamentary approval, the Children Bill will underpin this partnership-working with a duty for NHS bodies such as PCTs and Strategic Health Authorities to cooperate with other local services to deliver the *Change for Children* outcomes. The extent to which services are effectively joined up will also be considered as part of the new Joint Area Reviews of children's services.

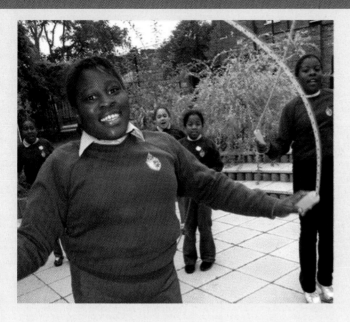

- childhood screening;
- immunisations;
- early interventions to address identified needs; and
- safeguarding children from harm.[6]

Immunisation

16. Immunisation is important in protecting individuals and population against disease which can kill or cause serious long-term ill-health. The UK's successful childhood immunisation programme means that childhood diseases (such as measles and meningitis C) are at very low levels, and some diseases (such as polio and neonatal tetanus) have virtually disappeared through the use of vaccines. It is the safest way for parents to protect their children against disease and the Government remains committed to maintaining an effective immunisation programme. However even where an area has high immunisation coverage certain groups of children may still be at risk. Health professionals therefore need to work together and ensure:

- access for vulnerable children and adults who remain unimmunised;
- that the needs of children and families with complex needs are met and services are tailored to meet their needs; and

- the organisation of services should include regular performance management with a focus on pockets of low uptake and areas of deprivation.

17. Children's trust arrangements will bring together planning, commissioning and delivery of children and young people's health services alongside education, social care and other partners, such as Connexions and (where agreed locally) Youth Offending Teams. **Children's trust arrangements will involve everybody working together locally to improve outcomes for children. The Government is recommending that all areas should have a children's trust by 2008.**

Integrating services

18. Children's centres are key to the integrated delivery of services through children's trust arrangements. **We will work with local authorities to establish up to 2,500 children's centres by March 2008. The Government's longer-term ambition is for there to be a children's centre in every community.** Children's centres are initially being developed in the 20% most disadvantaged wards – many children's centres are based on Sure Start local programmes.

---

6   Children's NSF – Standard 5: Safeguarding and Promoting the Welfare of Children and Young People; Paragraph 4: Impact that abuse and neglect have on children, pages 145–173. Published September 2004.
www.dh.gov.uk/PolicyAndGuidance/HealthAndSocialCareTopics/ChildrenServices/ChildrenServicesInformation/ChildrenServicesInformationArticle/fs/en?CONTENT_ID=4089111&chk=U8Ecln

CASE STUDY

The Manchester Family Link Workers Scheme, set up in July 2003, focuses on Harpurhey, the most deprived area in the country. It supports families with young children who have a wide variety of needs. The nine link workers were all recruited locally and spend a day a week studying NVQ Level 3 in health and social care and two days a week on placement with health professionals, including dieticians, midwives, speech and language therapists, health visitors, Sure Start workers and librarians. The remaining two days are spent supporting families, carrying out home visits, promoting primary healthcare and acting as the main link between families and Sure Start services locally.

The scheme has shown how multi-agency working tackles health inequalities, with North Manchester PCT working closely with the local Sure Start programme and the city council. Early signs are that the scheme is having a major impact on the uptake of services in the area, leading to the improved health of the community. The link workers' contracts run for two and a half years and all are optimistic that at the end of this period further opportunities will open up for them in the field of health and social care.

19. Children's centres bring together in one location a variety of services:

- ante- and post-natal care;
- routine and non-acute children's health services;
- child health preventative services;
- parental outreach and family support;
- good quality learning integrated with full day-care provision; and
- effective links with Jobcentre Plus, local training providers and higher education institutions.

20. The Child Poverty Review highlighted the importance of improving access to mental health care for children and young people. There is now evidence to demonstrate that the prevalence of mental disorders in young people has been slowly increasing, but provision for the mental health needs of 16 and 17 year olds often falls in a gap between services for children and those for adults. Self-harm in young women and suicide rates among young men are of particular concern. Child and adolescent mental health services (CAMHS) and adult mental health services need to work together more closely to ensure that arrangements at the interface between services properly take the interests and needs of young people into account. This will require services to be flexible in their approach in order to facilitate easier access to services and recognition of the importance to young people of being able to make choices

CASE STUDY

Ann, a health visitor in Leeds, leads a small public health team based in the children's centre. Her team has assessed the needs of the local population and has developed a series of initiatives that meet these needs.

The team is made up of a nursery nurse and two parenting facilitators. They use their available budgets to buy the services of a breastfeeding buddy from the local voluntary sector. The parenting facilitators support parents by running parenting groups at various sites throughout the community. The PCT sends out appointments to all parents when their first child is between two and three years old. This helps parents to manage their children's behaviour and to discuss how to give them the best start in life through healthy eating and lots of physical activity.

A few years ago the health visitor undertook a course in baby massage; she has now trained mothers from the local community to do this. The mothers now run classes for other mothers with infants where they can relax and chat for social support, and also learn techniques that improve how they bond with their babies. Mothers have found that their interaction with their babies has improved and their babies seem much happier.

about how and where their mental health care is delivered.

21. Another component of the strategy for integrated service delivery is the development of extended schools. **The Government's expectation is for all primary and secondary schools to develop as extended schools over time.** In partnership with PCTs and other agencies, extended schools can provide, or offer referral to, accessible health and social care to pupils, their families and the community. Extended schools can also provide opportunities for children and their parents to practice healthy lifestyles through opportunities for physical activity and classes, for example on cooking, outside school hours. One-stop shops and multi-agency health centres located on a school site enable health professionals to work alongside education and social care professionals, sharing both information and expertise.

22. The evaluation of the *Extended Schools Pathfinder Project* indicates that delivering health services in schools not only improves school attendance but gives health workers ready access to children and families who might otherwise not have attended clinics or doctors' surgeries.

Personal health guides for life

23. Chapter 1 set out as one of our key principles the importance of personalisation of support for

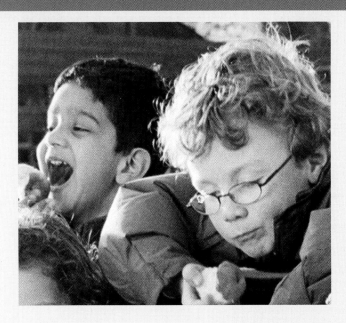

people to make healthy choices. We need to build a culture of participation where children and young people are involved in the range of issues and decisions that affect them. **We are introducing Children's Health Guides as part of the new** *Child Health Promotion* **programme. These health plans will be the foundation for personal health guides (PHGs) for life.**[7]

24. The health guide will encourage children and young people to build health into the way they live their lives. In a child's early life, the health guide, linked to and building on the child health record, will be developed and held by their parents or carers with advice and support from health professionals (including health visitors and school nurses). As they grow up, each child will take on responsibility for developing their own health goals with help from their parents, school staff and health professionals.

25. There will be opportunities to review plans at key transition points, such as starting school, moving to secondary school or starting work. Children and young people will get support to think about choices that impact on their health, and they will be encouraged to reassess their own progress towards good health and wellbeing.

Health visiting services

26. Health visitors bring specialist public health nursing expertise to integrated children's services, such as Sure Start and general practice. Their preventive work with families and communities helps parents to safeguard and promote the health and wellbeing of young children in areas such as healthy eating, preventing accidents and building effective relationships.

27. Health visitors will lead and oversee the delivery of the new *Child Health Promotion* programme and encourage the use of children's PHGs as part of family health plans. Working in children's centres, Sure Start local programmes and through links with local voluntary and community providers and general practice, they will deliver measurable health outcomes that focus particularly on vulnerable and disadvantaged children and parents such as teenage parents.

School nursing services

28. The Chief Nursing Officer's *Review of the Nursing, Midwifery and Health Visiting Contribution to Vulnerable Children and Young People*[8] emphasises the key role that school nurses can play, working with children and young people, parents and carers, teaching staff and others, to:

- review health at key stages and support development of children's PHGs;

7   Chapter 5 covers personal health guides for adults.
8   Department of Health, August 2004.

CASE STUDY

- provide general information, advice and support about health issues such as diet and nutrition, physical activity, emotional wellbeing, puberty, smoking and sexual health and about where to get further help and advice, including from Child and Adolescent Mental Health Services, social services and voluntary agencies; and
- support learning about health choices and managing risk.

29. We see a new and relevant role for school nurses on a wider scale than in recent years. **The Chief Nursing Officer will work with nurse leaders and the DfES to:**

- **modernise and promote school nursing; and**
- **develop a national programme for best practice that includes reviewing children's and young people's health and supporting the use of children's PHGs.**

In the North Tees and Hartlepool Trust area, there was a lack of structured, basic health education programmes for primary school children. The Trust therefore introduced a new school-nurse-led approach, stimulating children to take a positive interest in their health and in wider social and environmental issues as well as to build a sense of responsibility for their own health.

The project is a structured, basic health education programme for year 6 (10 to 11 year old) children and consists of six two-hour modules: accident prevention; personal hygiene; growing up; healthy eating; smoking/alcohol; and feeling good. It is recommended that a school nurse carries out the programme, alongside the class teacher, over one academic year.

Each module has an evaluation form in the resource pack. Feedback is encouraged from the school staff and children. The programme has now been offered to every primary school served by the Trust's school nursing service.

"I think there are things going on round here, but I don't really know about them, I think my friends used to go to a mother and toddler group, with people to talk to. Young kids are a handful, if there was one I'd love to go to it, but I don't think there is, I'm on my own here."

Listening to Children's Voices **research, 2003**

What can children, young people and parents expect from the school nursing service:
- to be involved in assessing their health needs and to be supported in caring and promoting their own health through PHGs;
- to have access to sensitive, confidential, expert health advice and support for their emotional wellbeing and health behaviours, including access to information through websites and text messaging;
- to have any health, medical and development problems identified and addressed in a way that minimises the impact of clinical conditions and disability on learning. The school nursing service will include:
  - appropriate training to support individual children with medical needs in school; and
  - to work with colleagues to ensure the school environment supports health improvement.

Cross-government strategy for tackling the root causes of physical and mental ill health in child abuse and domestic violence

Child physical, emotional or sexual abuse and neglect and domestic violence are causal factors in the mental and physical ill health of children, adolescents and adults and affect a significant proportion throughout their lives. The high costs in prevalence and economic burden on health and social care services and the criminal justice system have pushed these issues up the agenda.

They figure prominently in DH's policy on mental health, child health and women's health, and in wider government policy on child poverty, victims and witnesses, social exclusion and safeguarding children. They are also the focus of some cross-government working with DfES and the Home Office through the Inter-ministerial Groups on Domestic Violence and Sexual Offending in the wider context of new legislation on domestic violence, sexual offences and mental health.

CASE STUDY

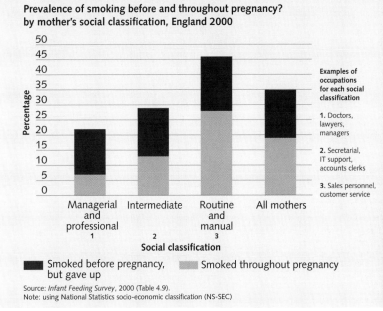

Prevalence of smoking before and throughout pregnancy? by mother's social classification, England 2000

Examples of occupations for each social classification

1. Doctors, lawyers, managers

2. Secretarial, IT support, accounts clerks

3. Sales personnel, customer service

Percentage

Managerial and professional 1   Intermediate 2   Routine and manual 3   All mothers

Social classification

■ Smoked before pregnancy, but gave up   ▨ Smoked throughout pregnancy

Source: *Infant Feeding Survey*, 2000 (Table 4.9).
Note: using National Statistics socio-economic classification (NS-SEC)

Parent to Parent, based at the Centre for HIV in Sheffield, trains parents to be volunteers who run sessions and one-to-one discussions with other parents and carers on how to talk to their children about relationships and sex. The aim of the project is to increase confidence and skills in communicating with children about sex, and to promote effective and consistent messages.

Parentline Plus runs the Time to Talk initiative, to encourage parents to talk to their children about relationships and sex. Time to Talk is supported by the Parentline Plus helpline and website.

30. We are providing new funding so that by 2010 every PCT – working with children's trusts and local authorities – will be resourced to have at least one full-time, year-round, qualified school nurse working with each cluster or group of primary schools and the related secondary school, taking account of health needs and school populations. School nurses and their teams will be part of the wider health improvement workforce described in Annex B. Roll-out will start from 2006–07 in the 20% of PCTs with the worst health and deprivation indicators.

SUPPORTING CHILDREN, PARENTS AND CARERS TO MAKE HEALTHY CHOICES

31. The new organisations for local delivery of services under children's trust arrangements will not focus on children and young people alone. Parents, both fathers and mothers, play a central role in ensuring that children get a healthy start in life. The *Choosing Health?* consultation made it clear that many parents want more support in this role and information about what they can do to make a difference. Parents and carers need access to reliable, consistent and easily accessible advice about how to support their children.[9] Individuals and families cannot provide this for themselves. Government and community organisations offer support to parents to carry out that responsibility.

---

9   Standard 2: Supporting Parenting, of the National Service Framework for Children, Young People, and Maternity Services.

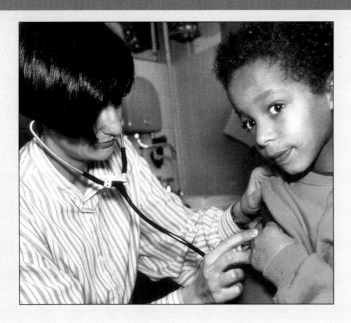

Information

32. Chapter 2 discusses what we are doing to make general information about health issues more widely available. **We will ensure that parents can access information and advice on their children's health through the e-Gov website and telephone lines and through links to Health Direct.**

33. We will also develop:

- **expanded support for parents, with targeted help accessible at key transition points in children's lives; and**
- **information for all parents on all aspects of growing up, delivered locally to best meet their needs through outlets in places such as children's centres, extended schools, libraries and GP practices.**

Support and advice

34. A key aspect of this work will be to support parents during pregnancy and in the very early years of parenting to break the cycle of inequalities between generations. The strategy to support parents in these early stages includes:

- continued support from maternity services and health visitors;
- improvements to public support on nutrition in the early years;

- improved support for learning and development in the early years; and
- Sure Start – which works to combat disadvantage in childhood.

35. The Government's national target to reduce health inequalities as measured by infant mortality by 2010 is already focusing action on improving services and support for pregnant women, new mothers and their babies.[10]

Maternity services

36. Good maternity services support parents, both mothers and fathers, before and during pregnancy, and after their child is born. Midwives provide advice about health and targeted care to mothers, fathers and their families. They have an important role in promoting health – helping pregnant women to stop smoking, improving nutrition and rates of breastfeeding, promoting mental health and building social support.

> The latest data confirm that children born to teenage mothers have the highest infant mortality rate of 7.9 per 1,000 live births (the rate is lowest for mothers in the 30–34 age group at 4.3 per 1,000 live births).
>
> ONS, Health Statistics Quarterly, Winter 2004

10 *Tackling Health Inequalities: A Programme for Action*
www.dh.gov.uk/PublicationsandStatistics/Publications/PublicationsPolicyandGuidance/PublicationsPolicyandGuidanceArticle/fs/en?CONTENT_ID=4008268&chk=Ad%2BpLD

CASE STUDY

In one of the most deprived areas of Liverpool a multi-disciplinary team of health visitors, midwives, GPs, pharmacists, Sure Start and a local PCT are invited to a two-day course to advise them on standardised techniques and signposting to encourage smoking cessation in all pregnant women and their partners. If this pilot is successful, the scheme will be rolled out to other areas in Merseyside.

One woman in four experiences domestic violence in her life, and this is associated with rises in the rates of miscarriage, foetal death and injury, low birth weight and prematurity. In the future, pregnant women will be routinely questioned by doctors and midwives during appointments early in pregnancy, such as foetal scans, about whether they have experienced violence at the hands of their partner. Those who require help will be referred to appropriate support and counselling services, or to the police if it emerges that they need protection or want charges to be pressed. Health service professionals play a crucial role in providing access to support mechanisms for women who are being abused. Using this infrastructure, it is hoped that women can be targeted at an early stage and abuse can be stopped before it escalates.

Nutrition

37. Nutrition is a key component of a healthy start in life and we are taking a number of steps to support healthy lifestyles for both parents and children.

38. **From 2005,[11] we will provide eligible pregnant women (including *all* pregnant women under 18), breastfeeding mothers and young children in low income families with vouchers that can be** exchanged for fresh fruit and vegetables, milk and infant formula[12] through a new scheme – *Healthy Start*. The scheme will be backed by a new communications campaign to help these families improve their diets and wider health, and make effective use of the vouchers. Infant formula milk will no longer be available from healthcare premises, which will reduce its promotion in the NHS.

39. Further action will include the review of Infant Formula and Follow-on Formula Regulations (1995) with a view to further restrict the advertisement of infant formula. **We will continue to press for amendments to the EU Directive on infant formula and follow-on formula.**

40. Health professionals will have a more visible role in the *Healthy Start* scheme, providing information and support to families on breastfeeding, child nutrition and other key health issues, including smoking and alcohol consumption. An important aim of *Healthy Start* will be to help health professionals to identify those pregnant women and young families who need extra support to make healthy choices. **A communications and training programme for health professionals will be introduced in parallel to the scheme and will be linked to the wider programme of support for staff described in Annex B.**

11 Once phase one has been completed in 2005, we will roll out the scheme nationally to around 800,000 families.

12 This replaces the existing *Welfare Food Scheme*.

CASE STUDY

As obesity and its effects are a real and current concern, Archbishop Sumner School set up the *Fit4kids* programme led by school nurses and that tackles any issues children have with food and exercise by providing exciting and fun after-school activities such as weekly exercise, cooking and gardening.

Parents are encouraged to participate by accompanying their child on a half-term basis, thus enabling the family as a whole to understand the issues around living healthily. *Fit4kids* has been extended to offer support to children from surrounding primary schools. One year 5 child has said, "it is great fun and I will learn about things to keep me healthy".

Supporting learning and physical and emotional development in the early years

41. The DfES's *Birth to Three Matters Framework (0–3)* and *Curriculum Guidance for the Foundation Stage (3–5)* support the provision of effective learning and development in the early years. They emphasise how crucial personal, social and emotional development are to very young children and are designed to give children the best opportunity for success in all areas of learning. More generally, they support development of physical skills and awareness of the benefits of being healthy and active, and the things that contribute to that such as sleep, hygiene, diet and exercise. Initiatives are already in place to drive forward these aims. For example, *Top Start*, a programme developed by the Youth Sport Trust, supports development of early movement and coordination skills in early years settings.

Sure Start

42. The Sure Start programme, launched by this Government in 1999 to improve outcomes for children, has already had a major impact in combating childhood disadvantage.[13] It has led a whole range of innovative developments to support the physical and emotional health of children and their parents in the early years, particularly those from the most deprived communities.

43. **The Sure Start Unit will put in place by late 2005:**

- **a training programme on social and emotional development to improve support for people delivering services for children between birth and age five;**
- **guidance for early years practitioners, focusing on changing patterns of parental behaviour and delivering activities that influence the physical health of babies and young children from conception to age five; and**
- **a *Community Parental Support Project* to promote greater parental involvement in children's early learning and development in some of the most disadvantaged areas. This will involve training four lead workers in each of the 500 communities supporting every Sure Start local programme, Early Excellence Centre and children's centre in England.[14]**

Other sources of advice

44. Parents often look to informal sources of help and advice. A wide range of voluntary organisations play an important role in supporting parents. For example, **Home Start[15] provides a home visiting programme with trained volunteers to support parents and families under stress in caring for and nurturing children during their early years. We have significantly increased funding to**

13 Five hundred and twenty-four Sure Start programmes have already been set up to increase the availability of childcare for all children, improve physical and emotional development in young children, and support parents.

14 Priority will go to training and support to health visitors and staff most likely to be in contact with families with very young children.

15 Home Start: Supporting families – Freephone National Information Line 0800 068 6369 www.home-start.org.uk

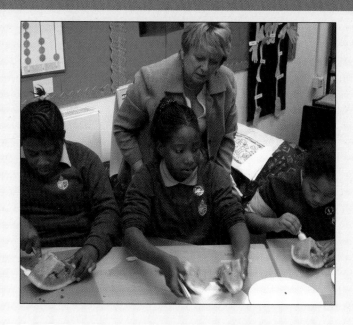

Home Start **so that by 2006/07 nine out of ten local authorities will have this service available.**

45. Parents will also be able to get more help and advice through the NHS to improve family health. Chapters 5 and 6 describe how NHS-accredited health trainers will offer personalised support to help people change their lifestyles and how all NHS staff will be better equipped to advise on healthy choices.

HEALTHY SCHOOLS – HEALTH AND EDUCATION GOING HAND-IN-HAND

46. Children spend on average a quarter of their waking lives in school. The school environment, attitudes of staff and other pupils, as well as what children learn in the classroom, have a major influence on the development of their knowledge and understanding of health.

47. The *National Healthy Schools Programme*[16] seeks to harness these opportunities by bringing policies and approaches that foster better health into everything that schools provide. **The Government has a vision that half of all schools will be healthy schools by 2006, with the rest working towards healthy school status by 2009.**

48. The *National Healthy Schools Programme* currently gives priority to improving children's health in the most disadvantaged areas. A recent

evaluation[17] shows that the programme is beginning to have a positive effect on health and wellbeing, particularly in deprived areas. Pupils in healthy secondary schools were, for example, less likely to have used drugs, had higher self-esteem, and were less likely to watch excessive amounts of television. In primary schools, pupils were less likely to be afraid of bullying. The evaluation also showed that Ofsted rated healthy primary and secondary schools as having better provision for Personal, Social and Health Education (PSHE), and pupils had more positive attitudes towards schooling. **We will encourage local *Healthy Schools* programmes to target deprived schools including Pupil Referral Units. We will also look to extend healthy schools to include nursery education.**

49. The results of the evaluation will inform the next phase of the *Healthy Schools Programme*. **From 1 April 2005, a healthy school will provide:**

- **a supportive environment, including policies on smoking and healthy and nutritious food, with time and facilities for physical activity and sport both within and beyond the curriculum; and**

16 www.teachernet.gov.uk/management/atoz/n/nhss/ and Healthy Living: the Blueprint.

17 Thomas Coram Research Unit/National Foundation for Education Research (2004) Evaluation of the Impact of the National Healthy School Standard – Research Summary. London: Thomas Coram Research Unit, Institute of Education, University of London/National Foundation for Education research. www.wiredforhealth.gov.uk/word/summary%20evidence%20+cru_nfer.doc

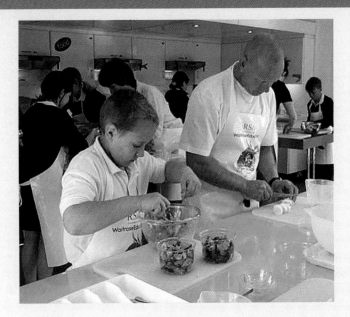

- **comprehensive PSHE.**[18] This includes education on relationships, sex, drugs and alcohol as well as other issues that can affect young people's lives, such as emotional difficulties and bereavement.

The *Healthy Schools Programme* will therefore focus particularly on key health priorities and will contribute directly to the delivery of national targets including those on childhood obesity and teenage pregnancy.

50. This new vision of healthy schools will be supported by the *Healthy Living Blueprint*. The Blueprint and supporting website[19] raise the issue of healthy living with both schools and early years settings and direct them to where they can access guidance, support and information.

51. These initiatives will be supported through the new approach to schools inspections that will be implemented by Ofsted from September 2005. Subject to parliamentary approval of relevant legislation, Ofsted will report on the contribution that every school makes to the five outcomes for children underpinning the *Every Child Matters: Change for Children* programme with increased emphasis on the health, safety and wellbeing of children and young people. These reports will be issued to parents and communities, identifying

where there are strengths and areas for improvement.

52. Ofsted is looking more widely at the contribution of education across children's health, drawing together evidence from across the curriculum, gathered by Her Majesty's Inspectors of Schools. It will also be conducting a review of the Physical Education (PE) School Sport Club Links strategy and the impact that educational provision has on pupil health and wellbeing.

53. **From 2005, all relevant inspections for services for children[20] will be carried out under a single overall inspection framework. This will focus on how services contribute towards improving the wellbeing of children and young people, including their physical and mental health.** New joint area reviews undertaken by teams drawn from several inspectorates will assess how, within a children's services authority area, services taken together improve children's wellbeing.

Food in schools

> 88% of all omnibus respondents think action to ensure schools only provide healthy meals would be effective.
>
> Opinion Leader Research

---

18 We will continue to support the roll-out of the PSHE Certificate Programme for teachers and community nurses in order that all schools are supported by PHSE specialists.

19 See www.teachernet.gov.uk/healthyliving

20 Including those by the Healthcare Commission, Commission for Social Care Inspection, Ofsted, Audit Commission and others.

CASE STUDY

St Thomas' is a small urban school with a higher than average number of children with caring responsibilities and children from transient families on roll. Learning Mentor, Deborah Stoker (a former Home Economics teacher), therefore established a Cookery Club with the aim of engaging with some children not accessing the full curriculum and with their families.

Every Tuesday afternoon, a small group of up to six children are taken off timetable for the last hour of the day and attend Cookery Club in the school hall. During the first hour, the children work with Deborah to prepare from fresh ingredients a simple healthy starter and pudding. Food safety and hygiene knowledge is developed, literacy and numeracy skills are reinforced and collaborative working encouraged. At the end of the school day, and for the second hour, the children are joined by their parents and carers. Deborah demonstrates a main meal. Everyone samples all the food and each family takes home the ingredients to make the main meal.

54. We are committed to developing approaches that take account of health in everything a school does. In terms of action on nutrition, that means we want to see all schools:

- deliver clear and consistent messages about nutrition and healthy eating;
- provide opportunities to learn about diet, nutrition, food safety and hygiene, food preparation and cooking as well as where food comes from; and
- actively promote healthy food and drink as part of an enjoyable and balanced diet and restrict the availability and promotion of other options.

55. Many schools have taken a fresh look at school lunches and have found that with a little creativity and enterprise they can provide attractive, nutritious meals that children enjoy eating.

56. **As part of the School Fruit and Vegetable Scheme, by the end of 2004 all four to six year old children in local education authority (LEA)-maintained infant, primary and special schools in England will be eligible for a free piece of fruit or vegetable every school day.** We are launching new materials and resources – including teaching materials, a video, a book, posters and a CD – to help schools integrate the scheme into the whole school approach to healthy eating and link to the 5 A DAY programme. Following evaluation, which

Children are increasingly being driven to school, rather than walking

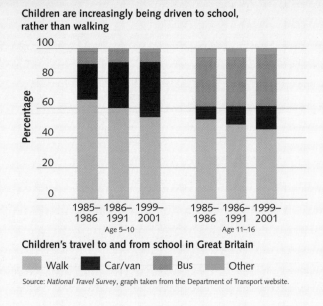

Children's travel to and from school in Great Britain

■ Walk ■ Car/van ■ Bus ■ Other

Source: *National Travel Survey*, graph taken from the Department of Transport website.

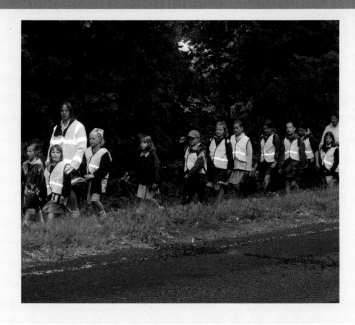

will be completed early in 2005, we will consider extending the scheme to LEA-maintained nurseries.

The scheme has had the most positive impact on younger parents (under 24 years) and parents from socio-economic groups C2DE. These parents have not only learned more than the other parents about the importance of eating fruit and vegetables, but they have also reported the highest increases in their consumption of fruit and vegetables at home.

57. We will invest over the next three years to improve nutrition in school meals by:

- **revising both primary and secondary school meal standards, to reduce the consumption of fat, salt and sugar and to increase the consumption of fruit and vegetables and other essential nutrients. We will strongly consider introducing nutrient-based standards. Ofsted inspectors will be looking at healthy eating in schools, and will take account of any school meals provided in doing so;**
- **subject to legislation, extending the new standards to cover food across the school day, including vending machines and tuck shops; and**

- **supporting schools to provide the best meal service possible – for example through new guidance on food procurement for heads and governors, and improving training and support for school meal providers and catering staff.**

This investment will enable schools to have more confidence in trying out new approaches and investigating whether they can build links with the local community, working with local providers and sourcing local produce.

58. The DH/DfES *Food in Schools* programme is assisting schools across England to implement the whole school approach to healthy eating and drinking. Over 700 local food partnerships have been established, where secondary school food specialists train their primary school colleagues in teaching diet, nutrition and cooking.

59. Following successful pilots in over 300 schools, a comprehensive *Food in Schools* package is being developed to support implementation of the whole school approach to healthy eating and drinking. Available from early 2005, this package will provide guidance and resources for schools to encourage, for example:

- **cooking clubs where children prepare and cook healthy food in a fun and enjoyable way;**
- **how to set up and manage healthy vending machines;**

CASE STUDY

Southend Borough Council introduced 'walking buses' in 1999 to enable children to walk to school safely and give children greater independence; there are now 24 operating in the borough. A walking bus lets a group or 'bus' of 15 to 20 children walk from home to school each morning guided by a 'driver' and a 'conductor', usually parents or volunteers, who pick the children up at predetermined bus stops along the way.

A sticker reward system is operated giving children the opportunity to claim small prizes for walking to school each day. Once a bus has been in operation for a year, the school receives a small grant of £1,500 to be used on green issues within their school. The service is promoted to children on the www.walkingbus.org website as a means through which they can spend time having fun with their friends before school, and to parents who are given advice on how to check if a walking bus route already exists for their children's school, and on setting up a new walking bus route.

CASE STUDY

Pupils at Oaklands Secondary School have been getting on their bikes in unprecedented numbers since it signed up to a travel plan. This was because of staff and parents' concerns over increasing traffic around the school, pupils' health and the contribution of the 'school run' to poor air quality and climate change. The school has seen over a 60% increase in cycling.

A mountain biking club was established, which also contributed to Oaklands' successful bid to become a sports college. City of York Council backed the travel plan by investing in secure cycle parking at the school and providing advanced cyclist training. Local cycle retailer, Cycle Heaven, provided pool bicycles for staff to use for short journeys during the day.

When asked her views on the travel plan as a pupil, Hannah Stone, aged 13, said, "The new bike sheds are much safer and there is much more room." Her classmate Ben Jameson added, "There are less cars than before so it is safer for everyone."

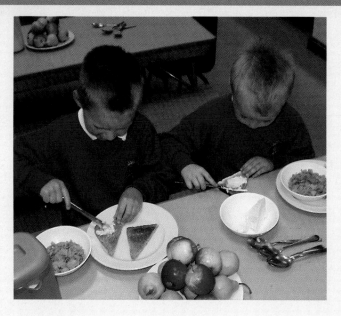

"There have been a lot of children coming through and asking for healthy lunches since the scheme was introduced."

"Some children have overcome a reluctance to eat fruit – often as a result of seeing their classmates enjoying it – while others were trying fruits they'd never eaten before."

"an excellent filler between breakfast and lunch, especially as certain children have little or no breakfast."

School Fruit and Vegetable Scheme participants

- **healthier breakfast clubs;**
- **tuck shops;**
- **lunch boxes;**
- **water provision;**
- **growing clubs; and**
- **the dining room environment.**

The package will be fully integrated into the *Healthy Schools* programme and supports the *Healthy Living Blueprint*.

Encouraging children to be physically active

60. Children's and young people's habits and their attitudes to physical activity impact on the choices they make later in life. We need to extend the opportunities that schools, working with local partners in the public and voluntary sector, provide through formal and informal opportunities for sport, play and active travel to and from school.

School travel plans

61. The number of children travelling to school by car has doubled over the past 20 years, with a corresponding decrease in walking and cycling to school. Rising car use on the school run contributes to congestion and pollution as well as reducing the likelihood that children will develop the habit of taking regular exercise.

62. We are encouraging more children and their parents to beat the traffic and improve their health

by walking or cycling to school through the *Travelling to School* action plan published last year.[21] *Travelling to School: A Good Practice Guide*[22] provides practical advice based on the many excellent school travel plans that already exist around the country.

> The contribution of the school journey to children's physical activity is important. Research by University College London showed that among the year 8 pupils sampled, more calories were burned up walking to and from school than during their two hours of weekly PE lessons.

63. **Building on existing progress, by 2010 all schools in England should have active travel plans. We are supporting the *Travelling to School* initiative by:**

- **funding around 250 local authority-based school travel advisers who are helping schools develop and implement travel plans; and**
- **providing small capital grants to help schools with an approved school travel plan to pay for items such as secure cycle parking and lockers.**

64. The School Transport Bill is designed to enable a number of local authorities to develop innovative school travel schemes. The Government expects local authorities applying to run school travel

21 www.teachernet.gov.uk/docbank/index.cfm?id=5154
22 www.teachernet.gov.uk/docbank/index.cfm?id=5172

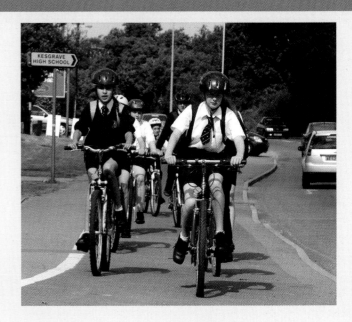

schemes to consider the travel needs of all pupils in their area. Each scheme will be tailored to meet local needs and priorities, but must aim to reduce car use and support measures to encourage pupils and parents to walk, cycle or take the bus wherever possible.

Support for children who want to cycle

65. Research suggests that after training, people cycle both more safely and more often. Cycling training in schools and communities across England is patchy, and while some local authorities run model schemes, others provide no training, or training on the playground only. Working with more than 20 road safety and cycling organisations, the Department for Transport has produced a new National Standard for cycle training. The Standard aims to ensure that trained children have the skills to cycle safely on the road.

66. We will drive forward action to implement the new National Standard for cycle training for children across England by 2005/06 by:

- establishing a formal cycle training and curriculum body – the Cycle Training Reference Group;
- funding instructor training schemes and accrediting existing training schemes and centres; and

- **providing a help desk and web database of trainers to support local authorities, schools and parents administer the National Standard.**

Physical education and sport

67. Research by the Qualifications and Curriculum Authority has demonstrated that using PE and school sport strategically makes a significant contribution to improving pupils':

- behaviour;
- attitudes to learning;
- attendance;
- engagement in healthy active lifestyles;
- standards in leadership and citizenship;
- inclusion in PE and sport; and
- attainment in PE and in subjects across the curriculum.

68. This is why **we are investing an unprecedented amount – in PE and school sport. The Government's national strategy for PE School Sport Club Links is the keystone of a bridge being built from PE to lifelong participation in sport via out-of-school-hours learning, inter-school sport and school–club links. DfES and the Department for Culture, Media and Sport (DCMS) will announce shortly funding they will make available in 2006–07 and 2007–08 to support school sport and the national strategy.**

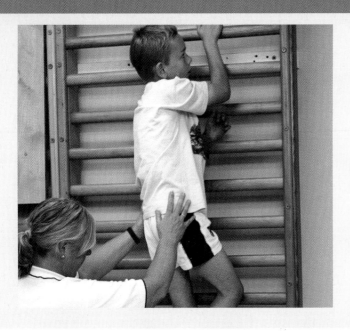

69. We are working through the PE School Sport Club Links strategy to ensure that continuing professional development programmes provide teachers with the knowledge and skills to:

- identify and support children who may be at risk from obesity; and
- work in partnership with the health sector to provide appropriate services.

70. Our national target, shared by DfES and Department for Culture, Media and Sport (DCMS), is to increase the percentage of schoolchildren spending a minimum of two hours each week on high-quality PE and school sport within and beyond the curriculum to 75% in 2006 and 85% in 2008. Currently, 62% of pupils in school sport partnerships meet the minimum requirement in a typical week.

71. Central to the strategy is the roll-out of school sport partnerships – families of schools that come together to widen and enhance opportunities for all their pupils, irrespective of their background and ability. **By September 2005, we will have increased by 33% (to 75%) the number of maintained schools (secondary, primary and special) in a school sports partnership and will achieve 100% coverage from September 2006. By 2006, we also aim to have at least 400 sports specialist schools and academies with a sports focus.**

72. We know that being in a partnership makes a difference. Evidence from the 2003/04 survey of school sports partnerships indicates that prolonged membership increases both curriculum provision of PE and overall participation in high-quality PE and school sport.[23]

73. School sport partnerships are required to ensure that all pupils benefit. For many partnerships this means offering a wider range of activities than before to engage those pupils who are not interested in 'traditional' team games. Over 40 sports are offered across all partnerships, and each partnership school provides an average of more than 14 different sports and activities. Dance, gymnastics and fitness are all popular. Many schools target provision at groups that are hard to reach or at risk of becoming disaffected. In particular, the Nike *Girls in Sport* project has had a real impact: 2,300 secondary schools (over 65%) to date have benefited from resources and training enabling teachers to rethink delivery of PE and sport in such a way that girls' interest is maintained.

74. Big Lottery funding is supporting each school sport partnership to set up a sustainable menu of out-of-school-hours learning opportunities. Many partnerships are using the funding to promote healthy lifestyles and physical activity as well as participation in sport.

---

23 The survey found that 68% of young people in those school partnerships that had been established for more than three years were participating in at least two hours of high-quality PE and school sport. This compares with those schools that had just joined the programme where 54% of young people were taking up their entitlement. Ofsted's second report on the programme (July 2004) confirms good progress and substantial improvements – particularly in terms of the quality of teaching – since their June 2003 report.

CASE STUDY

75. The Government is firmly in favour of competitive sport as a means of teaching teamwork, discipline, self-respect and how to cope with winning and losing. Increasing the quality and amount of competitive school sport is at the heart of our national strategy and is one of the key objectives for the network of school sport partnerships. In 2003/04, 96% of partnership schools held a sports day and 33% of pupils in partnership schools took part in inter-school competition.

76. Young people who see participation in sport and physical activity as something that only happens at school are more likely to give up once they leave. As part of the national strategy, we are supporting partnership schools to develop and strengthen links with community sports clubs to encourage participation beyond school. Through *Step into Sport* and *Club Links*, we are providing increased opportunities for young people to participate in community-based sport both as volunteers and as performers. More details of the Government's plans to provide access to sport through Extended Schools will be published shortly by DfES and DCMS.

77. The school sports strategy is making a significant contribution to our bid to stage the 2012 Olympic and Paralympic games. It is supporting and nurturing our most talented and

Bishop Challoner, serving a deprived inner-city area in Birmingham, has been a specialist sports college since 2000. The school has used specialist status and sport to raise standards. The percentage of pupils gaining five or more A*–C grade GCSE passes has risen from 37% in 1998 (well below the national average) to a staggering 76% in 2003. Provisional results for 2004 show another big increase with 85% of pupils gaining five good GCSE passes, well above the national average.

The benefits are being felt well beyond the school. In September 2003, the school setting became the hub of a school sport partnership – a family of 34 schools working together to enhance sports opportunities for all children. The 2003/04 school sport survey found that, after just two terms, the partnership was enabling 54% of its pupils to take up their entitlement to two hours of high-quality PE and sport each week. Funding from the *New Opportunities in PE and Sport* Lottery programme enabled the school to build a multi-purpose sports hall, a performance room and a martial arts dojo, which they share with other schools and the community.

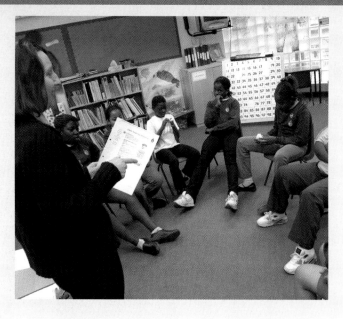

"To be able to meet friends in safe places."

"To get involved in more sports or physical activities, a wider range of activities, eg dancing, skateboarding, mum and daughter keep-fit, self-defence."

"Be involved in making decisions, eg on the local estate, or planning and delivering youth and health promoting activities or campaigns."

West Lincs PCT survey responses

gifted young athletes, some of whom will go on to compete at the 2012 games. Many of the volunteers being trained by *Step into Sport* will also be able to help with the increased demand for sporting activity generated through the bid to stage the games. Through *Dreams and Teams* and the *Global Gateway*, we are developing an international dimension to our network of sports colleges and school sport partnerships to foster world awareness.

78. Looked-after children and young people sometimes have particular difficulties in taking part in sports and leisure activities. The *Out of Hours Learning Project* is exploring the benefits to these children of being encouraged to take up sport as a hobby.

School playing fields

79. The Government has taken extensive measures to protect school playing fields. Legislation introduced in 1998 prevents schools from selling playing fields unless the land is surplus to the needs of other local schools and the community. **We are further strengthening the regime governing the sale of school playing fields by local authorities to ensure that:**

- **the sale of a playing field is an absolute last resort;**

- **as a first priority, sale proceeds are used to improve outdoor sports facilities; and**
- **new sports facilities are sustainable for at least 10 years.**

Developing emotional health and wellbeing

80. We know that children and young people who have good mental health learn more effectively. Emotional problems such as depression and anxiety and conduct problems have increased in children since the 1980s.[24] Deprived and abused children are more likely to suffer from mental health problems than average – for example behavioural problems have been found to be higher among homeless children. Although there is a strong association between emotional problems in childhood, teenage pregnancy and poor outcomes in adulthood, effective and timely interventions can reduce the incidence of serious health and social problems later in life.

81. The *Healthy Schools Programme* supports schools in developing an environment that promotes good mental health. We are evaluating the use of ENABLE – a CD-ROM designed to help schools identify and address the emotional health needs of children with emotional and behavioural difficulties – with a view to extending this model more widely.

24 *Time Trends in Adolescent wellbeing,* The Nuffield Foundation, 2004.

"Ban drinking on the street."

"Free or cheap leisure and sports activities designed by and promoted to young people, including more accessible services for young people with disabilities."

"For a teenager, the social benefits of risk-taking may well outweigh any perceived long-term consequences."

West Lincs PCT survey responses

CASE STUDY

82. We will continue to promote development of the skills that help children and young people make healthy choices through PSHE and Citizenship in school and the community. This explicitly supports emotional and social development and self-esteem, as well as developing key life skills such as assertiveness, conflict resolution, managing peer influence and peer pressure and identifying and managing risks.

83. A high proportion of looked-after children and young people have emotional and behavioural problems.[25] **We will publish guidance[26] next spring to help carers engage looked-after children in creative activity to improve their self-esteem, social skills and emotional wellbeing.**

84. The ethos and culture in schools impacts on all pupils. Anti-bullying has a high profile in the national key stage 3 Behaviour and Attendance programme and we are funding partnership working with key voluntary sector organisations to support anti-bullying work.[27]

SUPPORTING YOUNG PEOPLE IN SCHOOL AND BEYOND
Developing opportunities

85. The previous section set out some of the opportunities that children have to build up skills and understanding of what makes for a healthy life through their experiences at home, through

The MAC's programme has introduced multi-disciplinary teams into five schools in North Staffordshire to offer teenagers a one-stop shop to meet their personal needs, with another four schools planning to introduce them by spring next year and funding secured for a further five schools in the next financial year. The centres' professional health teams provide help and advice on issues such as alcohol, drugs, bullying and healthy eating as well as on relationships, sexual health and contraception.

The centres are generally open at lunchtimes throughout the school term on a drop-in basis, so no appointment is needed. As well as drop-in sessions, confidential advice is offered, including to those under 16 years of age, and this confidentiality aspect is very much emphasised to all pupils. Centre staff have been drawn from across the spectrum of health teams: from youth workers, school and 'Clinic in a Box' nurses, a local sexual health initiative, Connexions and Sure Start Plus advisers.

The programme is managed through the local Teenage Pregnancy Teams and receives funding from the four local PCTs of North Stoke, South Stoke, Newcastle-under-Lyme and Staffordshire Moorlands.

---

25 49% of looked-after young people aged 11–15 have a clinical mental disorder (Meltzer, H et al (2003) *The Mental Health of Young People Looked After by Local Authorities*. Office of National Statistics).

26 As part of the *wellbeing, Creativity and Play* project within the *Healthy Care Programme* for looked-after children and young people.

27 This includes the Anti-Bullying Alliance (launched June 2004), Parentline Plus, Childline in Partnership with Schools and the Diana Award.

CASE STUDY

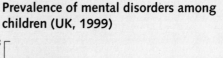

Prevalence of mental disorders among children (UK, 1999)

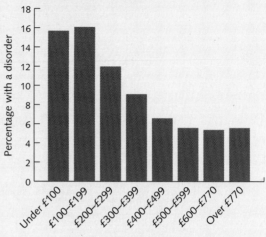

Gross weekly household income

Antenna Outreach in North London is helping African and African-Caribbean clients aged 16–25, who are socially isolated and have complex mental health problems, to participate in community life and to gain local acceptance by reducing the stigma associated with mental health.

Work placements, personal training, home tuition, short holidays and volunteering are offered as well as supported access to recording studios and sports facilities, medication and psychological therapies. The emphasis is on helping clients to develop social roles and explore the potential for independence rather than simple symptom reduction. Education and mentoring services are also available alongside traditional mental health services.

Clients are visited mainly between 9am and 5pm on weekdays, but there is also provision to see those who need extra social support at weekends. Users, their relatives and carers can contact a worker 24 hours a day via an on-call telephone. Clients report high levels of user satisfaction, particularly with regards to participating in the decision-making process, information about their treatment and understanding of their cultural needs.

interactions with their friends and at school. Adolescence is an important period of transition and a time when young people make many new lifestyle choices. Consistent support, clear boundaries and incentives can help young people to make positive choices as they gain independence.

86. Taking risks, experimenting and pushing boundaries is an important part of growing up. Young people need opportunities to learn about their world in ways that provide challenge and excitement through positive things to do and opportunities to play – as alternatives to experimenting with underage sex, smoking, alcohol and drugs. We need to help them understand and enjoy experimenting while minimising the risks of long-term damage to their health – accepting and understanding the responsibilities that go with choice in matters such as sexual behaviour.

There is a sharp increase in the prevalence of smoking with age – 1% of 11 year olds smoke regularly compared with 22% of 15 year olds.

The overall higher prevalence of smoking among girls than boys was found among all ages except age 11, where only 1% smoked regularly. For example, smoking was reported by 16% of 14-year-old girls and 26% of 15-year-old girls, compared with 9% of 14-year-old boys and 18% of 15-year-old boys.

Volatile substance abuse (VSA), the deliberate inhalation of volatile substances such as lighter fuel, glue or aerosols, is responsible for more deaths in young people aged 10 to 16 years in England and Wales than illegal drugs.

Sexually active under-16s are at particular risk of pregnancy and contracting sexually transmitted infection. They have high levels of regret and are the group least likely to use contraception.

87. The first step in influencing health behaviours in any group is to understand why people make the choices that they do. The second step is to design and deliver any new initiatives in consultation with them. Young people tell us that issues of smoking, drinking and sexual health tend to be presented from an adult perspective and do not fit the context of their lives or their experiences. Well-intentioned messages are either mistrusted or seen as irrelevant and about someone else. Young people do not consider the risks and benefits of different choices in the same way as adults.

88. **We are currently developing a new youth offer that will be the subject of a forthcoming cross-government Green Paper.** The offer will focus on creating the conditions for all young people to live healthy, happy, safe and prosperous lives and successfully make the sometimes complicated transition to adulthood. This will include specific new proposals to improve young people's mental and physical health and provide alternatives to risk-taking behaviour that has an adverse impact on health. It will start from the perspective of improving outcomes for all young people and will have at its core proposals that build on initiatives in this White Paper to:

- increase the choice and availability of opportunities for young people to engage in positive activities in their spare time, and to ensure there are places where they can be themselves and feel safe. This will include initiatives to encourage young people to access more physical and sporting activities;
- improve the relevance and accessibility of information, advice and guidance services that are available to all young people when they make everyday choices about lifestyles and

CASE STUDY

South Manchester PCT was one of 75 PCTs involved in the first national pilot of *Your Life!* magazine – an initiative designed to communicate key public health messages to younger women in disadvantaged groups.

South Manchester's edition of the magazine, produced in partnership with independent health information provider Dr Foster, focused on local priorities including breast cancer awareness, children's health, smoking cessation and sexual health.

The magazine represented a radical departure from traditional health communications and covered sensitive issues, particularly around sexually transmitted infections. Nevertheless, *Your Life!* won the support of Manchester's Chief Education Officer, Mick Waters.

Some 7,000 copies of the magazine were distributed through Manchester's secondary schools, attracting a positive response from both pupils and education professionals. South Manchester PCT's communications manager, Loren Grant, who led on the project, said, "It was not expected that all schools would welcome the way the magazine covered issues such as sexual health, but we were surprised by the positive response. We were also asked for extra supplies by some of our youth centres."

health – in particular smoking, drinking and sexual health;[28]

- build on *Every Child Matters* by ensuring that all young people are able to access expert advice and guidance when they need it – with a particular focus on those who are experiencing, or at risk of experiencing, poor outcomes because of mental health problems or substance misuse. This will include specific initiatives with groups who are traditionally hard to reach;[29] and
- develop new ways of supporting the parents of teenagers so that they feel equipped to help their children make informed choices, particularly on sensitive issues such as sex and relationships.

Targeting advice and support to young people

89. During adolescence, some young people, often those who are most vulnerable, may not attend school or access health services for advice and support. The youth service, *Young People's Development Programme* and outreach services have an important role in ensuring young people receive advice about health issues, particularly those who often feel excluded from services – such as those who are looked after, disabled or from black and minority ethnic groups, or from families who have experienced homelessness.

90. **We have funded a three-year *Young People's Development Programme* to pilot ways of**

---

28 Dedicated, accessible information and advice (for example, website information for teenagers) on sexual health and teenage pregnancy, and non-verbal communication techniques for some disabled young people. Modern communication routes such as text messaging, magazines and radio stations.

29 This means accessible services provided by adults who feel confident working with young people, for example youth workers, Connexions Personal Advisers, learning mentors and others who are equipped to offer basic health messages and understand when and how to refer teenagers on.

CASE STUDY

reducing teenage pregnancy and substance misuse and improving sexual health, particularly among vulnerable young people.[30]

91. The charity, SMARTRISK, runs an innovative *Heroes* programme warning adolescents about the risks of accidental injury and explaining how they can modify their behaviour to avoid such risks. We will work closely with SMARTRISK to assess the effectiveness of the *Heroes* programme approach in changing behaviour and how lessons might be applied in other programmes to improve health.

92. **We are supporting implementation of the Royal College of General Practitioners** *Getting it Right for Teenagers* **initiative, which provides a review checklist and training for GPs to help them develop services for young people.**

93. **We are developing a resource to support PCTs in making NHS services easy to use and trusted by young people.** *You're Welcome* **will be published early in 2005.**

94. **From 2006, the Department of Health will pilot health services dedicated to young people and designed around their needs. These services will include primary care and specialist services in locations that are aimed at attracting young people and will include facilities such as internet access.**

The Teenage Health Freak website, www.teenagehealthfreak.org, provides a wide range of information and advice about health issues for young people, such as stress, alcohol and other drugs, smoking, sex and relationships. It also gives answers to commonly asked questions and offers factual information on the range of health issues relevant to young people. The website is interactive and includes a range of quizzes and surveys that young people can do to check their knowledge about health.

There is also a virtual surgery where Dr Ann can be asked specific questions. Over 1,000 questions are sent to the site every month and a new question and answer goes on the site every day. Young people whose questions aren't answered get an automated response, based on a key word search, telling them where to look on the site and linking to information that is already available on the site. Over 1 million hits were received in July 2004, with teenagers staying online for an average of $10\frac{1}{2}$ minutes.

---

30 The programme is based on evidence from the USA demonstrating that intensive development programmes that meet certain criteria can improve young people's life skills, motivation and health-related behaviours. The programme is being extensively evaluated for possible wider development and to identify examples of good practice.

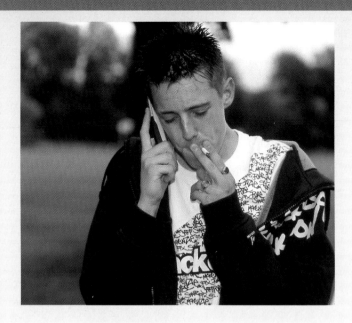

95. We are working with PCTs to pilot a new resource aimed at delivering health information for younger men aged 16 to 30. *FIT* magazine will be based on the *Your Life!* model, bringing together national and local content to reflect local priorities such as exercise, nutrition, smoking, alcohol, drugs, sexual health, violence and depression. *FIT* magazine will use the formats and techniques of lads' magazines to communicate health information to young men who are often hard to reach. A young men's editorial advisory board will be set up to work with the producers and advise them on how to ensure that the format is relevant and acceptable to the target audience.

96. We will ensure a broader reach of information about sexual health for young people in ways that they can access in complete confidence. This will include:

- confidential signposting to advice, plus easier access to 'teenage test your sexual health knowledge' material, to ensure all teenagers have access to the information they need at the time they need it;
- a confidential email service offered by trained sexual health advisers;

- provision of information via www.ruthinking.co.uk partnerships with specialist websites such as www.teenagehealthfreak.org and online youth portals;
- increased support for parents in talking to children about sex and relationships;
- provision of advice in settings where young people go;
- development of interactive learning material; and
- provision of targeted material for specific groups such as disabled children, young people in public care and care leavers.

Incentives for healthy choices

97. Choosing health will be harder for some than for others. It will be hardest when children and young people have experienced poor approaches to health while young, for those who have poor self-esteem and emotional health, and for those where risk-taking behaviours are already established. There is some evidence of incentive schemes being used successfully in the USA. They have also been used more recently in England, largely to reduce truancy and crime-related behaviour, and in Scotland to promote healthy eating among young people.

98. Such incentive schemes offer rewards to young people for adopting positive behaviours. **The**

CASE STUDY

The Karrot project is designed to help young people aged 11 to 16, living in the London Borough of Southwark, to feel safe, active and valued, to reduce numbers of young victims and perpetrators of crime, and to increase school attendance. Karrot offers sport, art, drama and music activities as well as a reward scheme for excellent school attendance each term, with special rewards to recognise improved behaviour and good citizenship.

The Karrot Internet Bus, containing state-of-the-art computers, synthesizers, software and broadband Internet access, tours schools, youth clubs, parks and estates around the borough. Special events are also organised to provide new and exciting experiences and challenges, including Kitch, a fashion show held at Tate Modern and attended by 1,000 people to showcase 10 young designers' winning collections. In its first year, the London Borough of Southwark saw youth-on-youth crime fall by 17%.

Department of Health has recently commissioned a review of the international evidence for incentive schemes. The aim is to assess which areas of public health could benefit the most and to consider some piloting work should the general approach look to be encouraging.

99. Through their national network of Connexions Partnerships, Personal Advisers are offering support on all aspects of young people's lives, including education, health, housing and employment, to some of the most vulnerable young people in England. Personal Advisers support the emotional and physical health and wellbeing of young people through offering tailored advice and support as well as effective referral to other services, and opportunities for play, creativity and recreation including sporting activities. Personal Advisers will be linked into the new local networks of NHS-accredited health trainers discussed in Chapter 5.

100. The Connexions Card is a secure smartcard available to all 16 to 19 year olds in England. The card enables young people to collect points for learning, training and development activities that can then be exchanged for rewards. **Connexions Partnerships and Learning Centres participating in the scheme can already award points to young people for progress in working towards an agreed goal or target. If the Learning Centres or Partnerships choose to, this can include rewarding**

positive health choices. We will continue to offer this facility and seek to encourage Connexions Partnerships and Learning Centres to link the card's reward opportunities with their other activities related to positive health choices.

Further educational settings

101. Young people need support as they go through the transition into adult life. **We will support the initiatives being taken locally by some colleges and universities to develop a strategy for health that integrates health into the organisation's structure to:**

- **create healthy working, learning and living environments;**
- **increase the profile of health in teaching and research; and**
- **develop healthy alliances in the community.**

PROTECTING HEALTH AND MANAGING RISK

102. While this chapter has focused on how we can provide support to children, young people and parents in making healthy choices, the Government also has a role in securing an environment that makes those choices easier. In some areas this means taking positive steps to protect children's and young people's health. Chapter 2 discusses the action we are taking on food, tobacco and alcohol promotion. We also need to strengthen action to tackle underage smoking and teenage pregnancy.

Underage tobacco sales

103. The Government is concerned about the number of children and young people who take up smoking. Too many children risk becoming addicted through buying tobacco illegally from shops. Much progress has been made recently on strengthening proof of age awareness among retailers through, for example, *Citizencard's* 'No ID/No Sale' campaign and the *Pass* (proof of age standards scheme) which is supported by all the leading retail trade associations. The scheme allows good proof of age cards to use their hologram logo which is difficult to forge. However, despite these excellent initiatives, there is evidence that illegal sales to young people under 16 continue to be a matter for concern.

- In 2002, 18% of children aged 11 to 15 tried to buy cigarettes from shops. Only 23% found that it was difficult to do so.
- Of children who tried to purchase cigarettes, fewer than half (48%) had been refused at least once.
- There were just 105 prosecutions in England and Wales for underage tobacco sales in 2003, with 84 defendants found guilty and 73 fined. Of these, just 11 fines were above £350.

CASE STUDY

Launched in 1995, the Health Promoting University initiative (HPU) is now well established within the University of Central Lancashire. It aims to promote the health and wellbeing of staff and students.

The 'touch' peer education and outreach project has been one of the most successful ventures, winning a North West Health Challenge Award. Launched in 1998, this is a multi-agency project focusing on safer nightlife issues, such as alcohol, drug rape and sexual health, with students trained to deliver outreach work within Student Union pub and club nights.

A number of resources specifically targeting younger students have been produced by the volunteers. Other key achievements include development by the University of corporate health and stress management policies and procedural guidelines on drug misuse, as well as the distribution of health handbooks for students and staff.

104. As part of our wider strategy, set out in Chapter 4, to protect children from exposure to smoke and smoking in restaurants, public houses and other leisure outlets, **we propose that legislation be brought forward to create new powers to ban retailers from selling tobacco products, on a temporary or permanent basis, if they repeatedly flout the law. This complements the work already under way to improve proof of age schemes. We intend to support this measure by looking at higher fines and updated guidance for magistrates, along with education for retailers on better compliance with the underage sales law. Before introducing these measures, we will consult with local authorities, the retail industry and other key stakeholders. We will support this with a communications programme for local authority enforcement.**

Teenage pregnancy

105. The Government's *Teenage Pregnancy Strategy* has two key goals: to halve the under-18 conception rate; and to increase to 60% the proportion of teenage parents aged 16 to 19 in education, employment or training by 2010. It aims to provide young people with the knowledge and skills to develop safe and responsible sexual relationships. The strategy has four themes:

- joined-up local action;

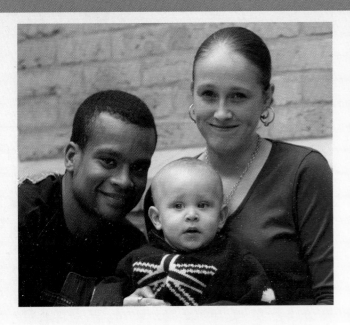

- a national campaign aimed at helping young people resist pressure to have early sex, raising awareness of sexually transmitted infections and encouraging the use of contraception and condoms by those who choose to be sexually active;
- better prevention through improved sex and relationship education in schools and community settings, support for parents in talking to their children about relationships and sex, and increasing access for sexually active teenagers to 'young-people-friendly' contraceptive and sexual health advice services; and
- support for teenage parents, including prevention of second unplanned pregnancies.

106. While the overall trend in teenage pregnancy is downward, in some areas of the country rates are level or increasing. Under-18 conceptions are highly concentrated, with the geography of 'hot spots' closely mirroring the pattern of deprived areas and low educational attainment. These 'hot spots' are distributed across England with the highest concentration in London. **We will support Teenage Pregnancy Partnership Boards to strengthen delivery of their strategy in neighbourhoods with high teenage conception rates.**

107. Choices for young people who become parents as teenagers are often limited in terms of continuing education, developing social networks and getting a job. This can lead to a loss of self-esteem and disadvantages for both young parents and their children. We are putting in place a range of initiatives to support teenage parents, including:

- *Care to Learn* – a programme designed to provide young parents with a focus for advice and support, and funding to provide for registered childcare and associated costs; and
- *Sure Start Plus* – a pilot programme to provide a coordinated package of support, including dedicated personal advisers, for pregnant teenagers and teenage parents. Evaluation has shown the benefits to young parents of having a dedicated adviser, including a significantly higher level of participation in education and training than the national average. The final evaluation of the programme will inform the most effective ways to improve outcomes for all young parents.

CONCLUSION

108. Actions in this chapter will build better opportunities for good health from birth to adulthood in all communities, and will provide all young people with the opportunities and understanding to choose healthy lifestyles by addressing inequalities.

- There will be new sources of information, guidance and practical support for parents, carers, children and young people themselves, provided in ways that are designed to meet their individual needs and be accessible to everyone.
- Services will be coordinated to meet the needs of children, young people and their parents and increasingly brought together in one location as part of integrated service delivery through children's trust arrangements.
- The components of good health will be a core part of children's experience in schools.
- There will be strengthened action to manage risk associated with underage smoking and sexual activity.

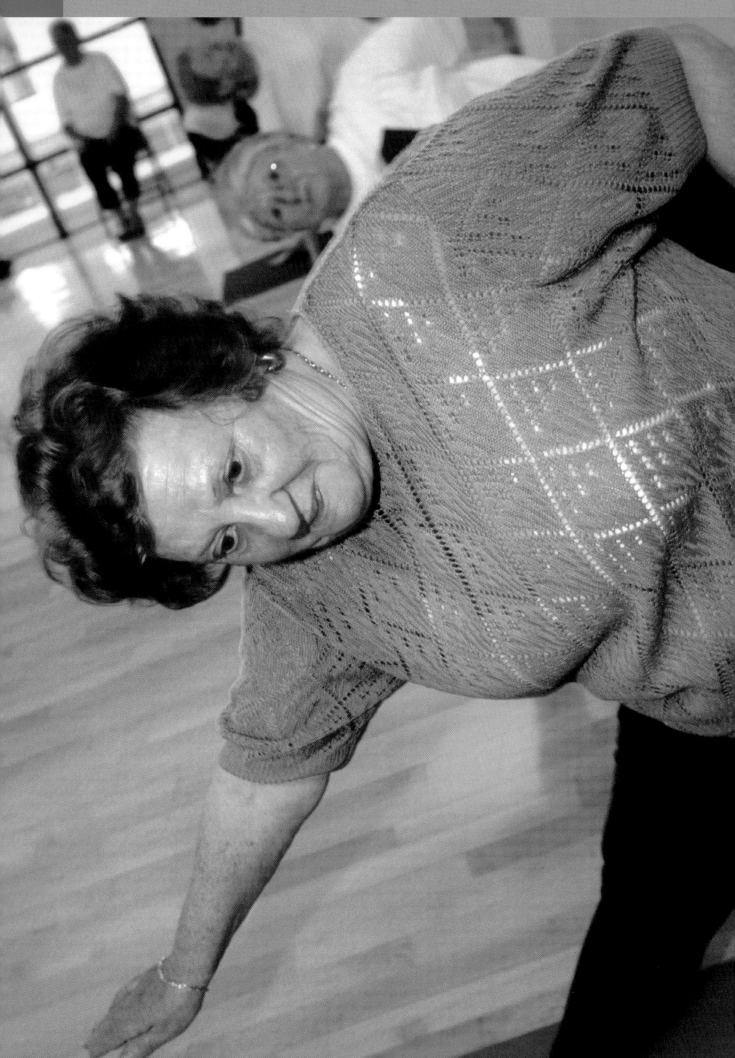

CHAPTER SUMMARY

The environment we live in, our social networks, our sense of security, socio-economic circumstances, facilities and resources in our local neighbourhood can affect individual health.

There are unacceptable differences in people's experience of health between different areas and between different groups of people within the same area. Action by local authorities working with local communities, businesses and voluntary groups to tackle local health issues makes a difference to the opportunities for both adults and children to choose healthier lifestyles. This chapter sets out action to maximise the positive impact of the local community setting with measures that include:

- *local authorities providing local leadership to bring concerted and integrated local action on health;*
- *investment and new initiatives in disadvantaged and deprived communities; and*
- *promoting partnership between the public and voluntary sectors with business to develop national and local champions for health and extend opportunities for people to take up healthy lifestyles in local communities.*

Smoking is a major cause of ill-health. Balancing the rights of people who choose to smoke against the interests of the majority who object to being exposed to second-hand smoke at work and in public places was one of the most controversial issues in the consultation. This is an area where campaigns and public demand for change have not done enough to achieve national targets to reduce prevalence in smoking. We therefore intend to shift the balance significantly in favour of smoke-free environments.

By 2006, all government departments and the NHS will (subject to limited exceptions) be smoke-free. We will consult on detailed proposals for regulation with legislation where necessary so that by the end of 2008, all enclosed public places and workplaces will be smoke-free except those specifically exempted.

INTRODUCTION

1. Our health and the lifestyle choices we make are affected by where we live, our personal circumstances, and relationships with the people around us.

2. Well ordered and stable communities, with good access to services, clear leadership, cohesion and strong partnerships between local government, business, the voluntary sector, health services and community organisations provide an environment

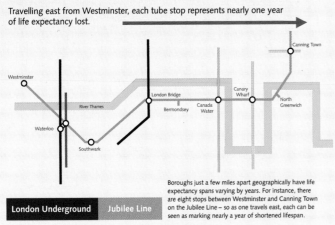

Differences in life expectancy within a small area in London

Travelling east from Westminster, each tube stop represents nearly one year of life expectancy lost.

Westminster

River Thames

Waterloo

Southwark

London Bridge

Bermondsey

Canada Water

Canary Wharf

North Greenwich

Canning Town

Boroughs just a few miles apart geographically have life expectancy spans varying by years. For instance, there are eight stops between Westminster and Canning Town on the Jubilee Line – so as one travels east, each can be seen as marking nearly a year of shortened lifespan.

London Underground   Jubilee Line

Source: London Health Observatory based on Office for National Statistics data.

that helps people make healthy choices. Divided communities with high crime rates, inadequate or disjointed services make it harder to be healthy. The stark postcode divide in health expectations between neighbouring communities is evidence of that. But that divide also makes clear the opportunities at a community level for making very significant differences to the health of local communities.

3. Clearly individuals on their own cannot change their local environment. That must be the work of local government and local voluntary and community organisations. The health inequalities between localities makes obvious the opportunities at a local level for making very significant differences to the health of local communities. Often these issues seem intractable – they take time, imagination, money and sustained leadership through committed partnerships to overcome. Success in tackling the health challenges we face requires measures to support the development of the social and organisational community infrastructure that empowers people to make healthy choices. This can only be achieved through collective action.

4. Nationally this needs to be a cross-government strategy that empowers local government, local NHS and community organisations to take action to improve health at community level through:

- supporting communities' own action;
- local authorities providing local leadership;
- partnership working: NHS primary care trusts working with local authorities and others (including the voluntary and community sector) to tackle inequalities and respond better to what people want and need, prioritising action where it will make most difference;
- corporate social responsibility: organisations promoting health both as employers and as producers; and
- regulation of smoking in the places where people come together for work, activities and leisure.

IMPROVING HEALTH – THE POTENTIAL OF COMMUNITY ACTION

5. Individuals belong to a range of overlapping communities – their local neighbourhood or estate, a faith or age group, communities relating to common interests or social networks such as sports clubs or work networks. Some will be informal groups, while others will be more formally recognised within the public sector and may already be involved in specific programmes or initiatives to promote health. Many of these can provide support for individuals who are trying to make more healthy choices through opportunities that they cannot provide for themselves.

CASE STUDY

6. Communities are vital in improving health and can play a significant role in promoting individual self-esteem and mental wellbeing and reducing exclusion. Help and encouragement from friends, neighbours and work colleagues can make a significant difference in ensuring that individuals feel supported in making positive choices about their lifestyles. It is easier to quit smoking, breastfeed your child, and exercise regularly with the encouragement and support of people around you.

7. Voluntary sector and community organisations are often much better than the statutory sector at engaging with groups of people who face most difficulties or who do not access traditional sources of advice on health. For the public sector, working in partnership with community organisations provides the opportunity to learn from the skills that community activists use.

8. Community organisations can increase opportunities for healthy choices, for example through setting up food co-ops or through action for safe parks and streets so that people can exercise safely. There are a growing number of green gyms – schemes that support people in gardening or local environmental improvement while providing opportunities for exercise and developing social networks. Social enterprises – businesses with a social purpose – also make a positive impact on the health, wellbeing and

The award-winning Healthy Heart project was established to tackle one of Hyndburn and Ribble Valley's leading health problems, coronary heart disease, and to prevent the social isolation of certain community members. The project team identified a derelict community allotment and renovated it into a resource that the community uses to grow fruit and vegetables and to promote biodiversity. The project has improved the physical, social and mental health of participants by providing opportunities for increased physical activity and healthy eating, as well as engendering a sense of ownership.

Relationships have also been built with other local organisations, including Learning Disabilities, a number of schools, and Bootstrap Enterprises, a charity which assists individuals with re-entering employment. As a result of the latter, two clients now have individual plots to grow their own food. In addition, five training programmes have been set up to develop skills, including visits to other local horticultural sites, with the aim of making participants more employable.

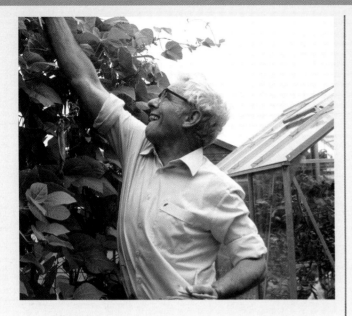

CASE STUDY

prosperity of communities. Services provided at a community level, and involving the community, are often the most effective way to improve health. All of these activities are beyond the capacity of individuals and their families but they demonstrate how collective action can improve the environment for health.

9. The Government is promoting new approaches that involve communities and extend the power of individuals to act within communities – engaging with families and communities where they are. The skills, know how, social networks, motivation, resilience, tradition and culture that exist within communities can be a powerful force for promoting and protecting health. Increasingly, new services are being delivered through community-based initiatives like extended schools, Sure Start local programmes, children's centres, the Healthy Communities Collaborative and the Expert Patients Programme.

10. 5 A DAY community initiatives in deprived areas, funded with £10 million from the lottery, are currently delivering a range of activities in 66 primary care trusts (PCTs). The initiatives aim to improve access to fruit and vegetables, increase awareness of their health benefits and increase consumption, with emphasis on addressing inequalities. Activities include advice in primary care on how to incorporate fruit and vegetables into the diet, home delivery schemes,

The Healthy Communities Collaborative is a programme run by the National Primary Care Development team, involving local people and professionals from a range of agencies and voluntary bodies, who work together to effect change on a health-related subject.

The original topic, which was piloted in three areas across England, was reducing falls in the over-65 age group. The work resulted in a drop of 32% in the number of falls recorded by ambulance collection data during the one-year pilot. Older people and professionals worked to minimise personal and environmental risk in simple and practical ways, employing evidence provided by the Health Development Agency. The pilot has now spawned eight other sites, which have put into action best practice in this area.

The original three areas have gone on to address some of the issues associated with healthy eating. Teams have already set up breakfast clubs for children, engaged a mobile shop to make stops selling fish, fresh fruit and vegetables in an area with no local outlet for fresh food. They have also worked with the Co-op and Sure Start to provide 300 hand blenders to mothers with babies reaching weaning age, once they have completed a three-week course on weaning babies the healthy way.

CASE STUDY

Manchester Community Sports Development runs sport and physical activity programmes which put young people who are at risk, and/or causing youth nuisance, through accredited training programmes in Central ward. These are run by Manchester Leisure, predominantly during the twilight hours from 6pm to 9pm, which have been identified as key youth offending times. They are delivered through existing Community Sports and Youth Offending Team Networks. During its first year, 1,488 young people participated in the programme, with 27 young people gaining a nationally-recognised sports qualification. Four young people trained to become coaches and a similar number became qualified Level 1 football coaches. One young person completed and passed the RLSS Swimming Award.

development of better cooking and gardening skills and setting-up food co-operatives.

11. Evaluation of the five early pilots, funded by the Department of Health, showed that over a year, the community initiatives had increased average consumption of fruit and vegetables by one portion a day among those people with the lowest intakes. **The Department of Health is committed to funding similar community food initiatives, following evaluation of the lottery-funded pilot initiatives, in more PCTs from 2006. The focus will be on deprived communities and will build on the lessons to come out of the evaluation of lottery-funded initiatives.**

12. To support the work at the local level, new resources will be launched in early 2005 to help healthcare professionals support people to increase their fruit and vegetable consumption, including a short 5 A DAY questionnaire to assess consumption levels. These resources are also useful when giving general advice on diet and nutrition and will support work on obesity prevention and management.

13. Extended schools working in partnership with local bodies (PCTs, social services or as part of a cluster of schools) can provide integrated services to the whole community. These might include:

- breakfast clubs, encouraging a healthy start to the day;
- counselling services;
- opening up access to sports and leisure facilities after school hours;
- family support, for example, healthy cooking courses;
- ante- and post-natal classes;
- NHS Stop Smoking sessions;
- first aid training;
- health advice for young people; and
- primary care provision.

14. The Healthy Communities Collaborative on falls prevention empowers local communities to deliver change for themselves. Championing social inclusion, providing social support and using team building in a 'plan do study act' cycle it achieves change that professionals alone are unlikely to achieve. It has now extended beyond its original focus to a broader health improvement focus; it creates partnerships that might not otherwise exist between a broad range of players and helps professionals to realise what can be achieved through community action. Supporting community action is central to this White Paper. **We will extend the current healthy communities collaborative to more deprived communities from 2006, and we will use collaborative techniques to support action through local partnerships (see also Chapter 6).**

15. We are working with the NHS, voluntary and community sectors to support a stronger role for community-based organisations in delivering NHS and social care services. **Working with the new**

National Strategic Partnership Forum from November 2004, we will encourage activity to promote health through co-operation and partnership between the NHS and the voluntary sector and link this into the specialised public health *Phorum*,[1] which will also be strengthened.

16. Local people and local services often identify poor health and health inequalities as being at the heart of wider problems such as educational underperformance and chronic unemployment within their area. Poor health is often compounded by other problems such as poor housing, poor quality street environments, and inadequate transport and leisure provision. Living in a safer environment extends opportunities for people to be physically active and develop social networks – feeling safe helps people choose health. Improving health can also have a positive impact in reducing crime and disorder, particularly where problems are associated with alcohol, drugs or violence.

17. The Government's Neighbourhood Renewal Strategy recognises the links between different issues, and is focused on working with communities to improve outcomes in the most disadvantaged areas. The strategy focuses on five themes: improving health, education, housing and the physical environment, and reducing crime and unemployment. Extra funding has been made available to the most disadvantaged local authority areas, and part of this is being used to support work to tackle health inequalities and resolve underlying causes of decline where they exist.

18. **We will publish revised guidance on health and neighbourhood renewal, early in 2005, to support local action to address health inequalities and deliver neighbourhood renewal.** The guidance will complement the measures outlined in this White Paper and offer practical support and help to local authorities, PCTs and other players in using available resources and information flexibly to focus local action on reducing health inequalities.

NEW FORMS OF COMMUNITY VOICE AND ACTION – COMMUNITIES FOR HEALTH

19. We also want to encourage new forms of community leadership. **We shall work, initially with 12 localities, to pilot a new approach to unlocking the energy that lies within communities themselves. *Communities for Health*, beginning in Spring 2005, will promote action across local organisations – voluntary sector, NHS, local authorities, business and industry – on a locally-chosen priority for health, to celebrate current achievements, and build momentum for future change.[2]**

---

1   The *Phorum* is an official Government initiative sponsored and chaired by the Department of Health, and developed and managed by the Health Development Agency, with a steering group of non-governmental public health organisations actively contributing to it. Collectively it works to support engagement between Government and different non-Governmental organisations (NGOs) on health inequalities and wider public health issues.

2   In the first year of *Communities for Health* we shall issue invitations to areas which can demonstrate a strong basis of partnership working and action on health inequalities. The DH will provide central coordination, support materials and marketing, and project funding. Local partners will develop and manage programmes. They will identify their biggest local health challenge or the one where there is most potential for movement, and look at ways of maximising community support and action for change. This will involve local government and the NHS finding new ways to join with community leaders, employers, local chambers of commerce, the media, voluntary sector partners, plus informal community groups and organisations.

'An annual report about the state of people's health and of the major determinants of health should be made available at national and local authority levels to encourage understanding.'

Derek Wanless, February 2004

Difference in years between lowest and highest life expectancy within selected boroughs

Borough	Lowest ward level life expectancy	Highest ward level life expectancy	Difference (years)
Westminster male	67.4	82.6	15.3
Westminster female	72.2	86.4	14.3
Camden male	69.5	79.6	10.1
Croydon female	76.4	87.1	10.7

INFORMATION FOR LOCAL COMMUNITIES

20. If local communities are to take action to improve health, they need clear, understandable and timely information about local needs and trends. In Annex B we discuss the wider role that Public Health Observatories and Regional Directors of Public Health have in surveying health and providing data to support local action to promote health.

21. PCT Directors of Public Health are already expected to publish annual public health reports, highlighting local health concerns and making recommendations for action. Local partners, particularly the PCT and local authority, should respond formally to these reports, setting out the actions they intend to take and progress against previous years' recommendations. Local Scrutiny Committees have a role in reviewing their plans on behalf of the community.

22. We believe there is more to do, to ensure that all communities benefit from clear, accessible information that sets out progress on health locally, so that people can understand the issues and engage in action to improve health in their local communities. **We will develop a standard set of local health information that can be linked to other local data sets for publication. Public Health Observatories will produce reports designed for local communities at local authority level[3] which will support Directors of Public Health in**

promoting health in their area. The first of these local reports will be published in 2006 and we will also publish the first national report that year. These reports will include specific information on different groups in the population, for example on black and ethnic minority groups, where available.

Community leadership for wellbeing

23. Local authorities have a responsibility to provide community leadership in the areas they serve. This includes a specific legal power to promote wellbeing (Local Government Act 2001). They are well placed to promote understanding within local communities of how good health and reducing inequalities can have a positive effect on the local economy, social and environmental fabric. They have the lead responsibility for social care and for scrutinising health arrangements in their local areas. Their contribution extends across planning, housing, the local and built environment, transport provision, fire safety, environmental health – for example air quality issues, trading standards, education, childcare, leisure, and services for people with disabilities and for older people.

24. At a local level, securing healthy communities depends on PCTs working closely with local authorities and other partners through Local Strategic Partnerships. The best Local Strategic Partnerships have been very effective in bringing

3   These reports will bring together information for neighbourhoods on the basis of local authority boundaries, supplementing existing Director of Public Health reports with consistent national reporting of key data, which will become available over time, on areas such as levels of exercise, smoking and nutrition – so that everyone is able to follow trends, and compare local progress against similar areas.

CASE STUDY

Fit for the Future is a long-term strategy, launched in October 2003, which has helped to reduce large-scale health inequalities in Barnsley. All the key local agencies and sectors are signed up to the strategy, which is embedded within the role of the Local Strategic Partnership. Activities include stop smoking services with young people, a 12-week weight management programme, an initiative to reduce fuel poverty, and a welfare rights benefit advice service within GP practices. A 'Champions Award' has also been developed to celebrate the achievements of local people and groups.

The strategy has been supported by a social marketing and communications campaign to fully engage the community, increase awareness about health inequalities and raise the profile of the programme.

---

about real improvement in the health of their communities by facilitating joined-up planning and delivery. Strong leadership through Local Strategic Partnerships, with direct involvement from PCT chief executives and other senior NHS representatives, is often the key to success in a joined-up approach to health improvement.

25. Many health partnerships which sit within the Local Strategic Partnership structures have built on the successful work already established by *Healthy Cities*, *Health Action Zones* and *Health Improvement Plans*. The most successful approaches to improving health and tackling health inequalities are based on effective engagement of communities, through the Local Strategic Partnership and arrangements that:

- bring together needs assessment, planning and commissioning processes across different sectors – such as housing, health, planning, child and social care;
- are based on common local targets and indicators of success;
- use resources flexibly and ensure that inequalities are targeted and tackled effectively; and
- are supported through joint appointments, including a joint Director of Public Health.

Local Area Agreements

26. The Government gave a strong emphasis to the importance of local partnership working through Local Strategic Partnerships. But in the past the way that individual initiatives have been set up to address different problems in different areas has often led to many separate funding streams, each with different processes and conditions attached.

27. To make Local Strategic Partnerships even more effective we are introducing new Local Area Agreements. **Working with local government and other partners, including PCTs and children's trusts, we will pilot Local Area Agreements in 21 areas, starting in April 2005. If the pilots are successful, agreements will be rolled out nationally. Local Area Agreements will be based on agreements between Government, councils and local partners about local delivery of national targets in ways that reflect local priorities, reinforce joint working between partners and make more flexible use of central government support, bringing together different funding streams to best meet local priorities.**

28. The Department of Health and the NHS will work with Government Offices for the Regions to develop effective arrangements to help councils and their partners develop Local Area Agreements that improve health.

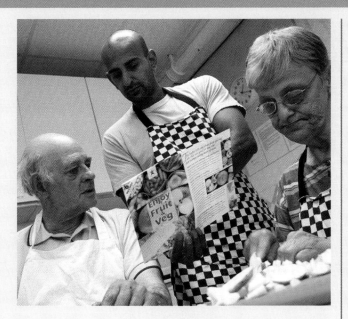

CASE STUDY

Supporting People programme

The Supporting People programme, which provides housing-related support to vulnerable people, plays a key role in supporting public health delivery through helping people to develop or retain the skills needed to maintain independent living. The positive impacts of the programme can include preventing admission to hospital, assisting and facilitating discharge, and helping to develop the skills needed to maintain a healthy lifestyle.

The programme is administered at a local level by the 150 top-tier (ie county and unitary) local authorities, who commission and manage housing-related support services based on local needs and priorities through partnerships with Probation and PCTs. The latter have a key role to play in ensuring that local Supporting People services complement local relevant care and health services, so that they support health as well as housing objectives and targets.

29. **From 2005–06 onwards, we will require PCTs to develop targets to meet the needs of people living in their area that are agreed with local partners and designed to meet national targets and priorities set by this White Paper and the NHS Improvement Plan.** These local targets will need to:

Lizzie is a client of Revolving Doors Agency's Islington Link Worker Scheme. She has a long history of alcohol abuse and is well-known to Islington police, having been arrested on numerous occasions for being drunk and disorderly and for aggressive begging and common assault. She lost custody of her children and lost her local authority flat following a fire. She has been homeless since then.

Revolving Doors' work with Lizzie demonstrated that she was much more mentally vulnerable than her psychiatric assessments suggested and was unable to care for herself. Her cognition and functioning appeared to be deteriorating and she was consistently confused, anxious, disorientated and unable to manage her basic needs, such as hygiene and nutrition.

Through joint work with Camden Social Services, the resettlement worker at her shelter and the Rough Sleepers Initiative workers in Camden and Islington, the Link Worker team helped Lizzie to access a long-term placement at a 'wet' Registered Care Home. For the first time in many years, she has a permanent address and access to high-level, consistent support. Since then, the Link Workers have not seen Lizzie on the streets or in the police station.

- address local service gaps;
- deliver equity by targeting groups and areas with the worst health outcomes;
- be evidence-based;
- be developed in partnership with other NHS bodies and local authorities; and
- offer value for money.

This will enable PCTs to play a strong part with other local partners in action on Local Area Agreements and other locally agreed plans.

30. To support the development of local data sources, and improvements in data quality, the Department of Health will continue to work closely with the Department for Education and Skills to develop appropriate systems for recording lifestyle measures, for example obesity through weight and height measurements, among school age children.

PROMOTING PHYSICAL ACTIVITY THROUGH COMMUNITY ACTION

31. Many people are looking for ways to fit more physical activity into their lives. This is vital if we are to reverse the rising incidence of obesity. But often people face real and perceived obstacles to doing as much as they would like. They tell us that they want more access to high-quality green spaces, to be confident they can walk safely in local streets, to have more routes designed with cyclists and pedestrians in mind, and more affordable access to swimming pools or gyms.

CASE STUDY

The Shared Priorities project builds the capacity of local authorities to enable them to work with PCTs and regional partners to promote healthier communities and narrow health inequalities. Twelve authorities are already signed up to the project.

The Safer Communities Shared Priority is one of four work streams currently underway, along with educational attainment, improving the local environment and reducing health inequalities. In the deprived area of Chester-le Street, car crime has been reduced by nearly 20% in the last year, and domestic burglary by approximately 37%, thanks to a number of initiatives including a harm reduction programme in the local Civic Centre by a PCT partnership. This has been helped by the area's Education Resource in Communities bus (known as ERIC), a fully equipped mobile youth and community centre that provides health and drugs information, and development and leisure activities in areas that are without adequate provision.

'A mass shift in current activity levels is needed. This will only be achieved if people see and want the benefits but also if opportunities are created by changing the physical and cultural landscape – and building an environment that supports people in more active lifestyles. If people of all ages can be engaged in a new way of thinking about active lifestyles, better health can be a realistic goal for all.'

Chief Medical Officer's report on physical activity[4]

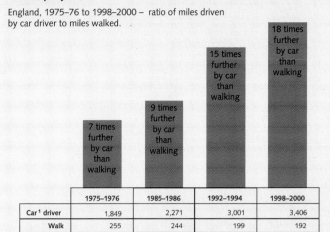

Average distance driven in a car* in relation to distance walked per year

England, 1975–76 to 1998–2000 – ratio of miles driven by car driver to miles walked.

	1975–1976	1985–1986	1992–1994	1998–2000
Car[1] driver	1,849	2,271	3,001	3,406
Walk	255	244	199	192

'Car – driver' and 'Walk' are two of sixteen modes of travel detailed in the National Travel Survey.
* 'Car' includes 'light van'.
Source: National Travel Survey 2002

32. Limited access to opportunities for exercise can be a significant cause of health inequalities. Older people may feel unable to walk in their neighbourhoods because of the state of the pavements, a poor level of street lighting or a fear of crime. Adults in residential homes may be significantly disadvantaged in accessing opportunities for physical activity. People of all ages are discouraged from walking or cycling by excessive traffic and its speed.

33. Poor-quality local environments also have wider impacts on public health. Fear of crime and poor maintenance can stop the use of children's play areas. Air pollution will trigger asthma attacks and cardiovascular problems. And poor-quality housing has been clearly shown to have detrimental health impacts.

34. Opportunities are well placed to increase opportunities for physical activity in partnership with the independent and voluntary sector. Alongside their general powers they have specific functions in relation to leisure facilities, school sport, parks and open spaces, planning and transport and the maintenance of public rights of way and footpaths in town and country and the provision of recreational opportunities in the wider countryside. Local cultural strategies include plans for sports and recreation and create opportunities for groups of people who are not traditionally

engaged in exercise to become active. They provide the opportunity to build a diverse range of facilities and venues to reach a wide range of people of all ages. Leisure and culture providers – including pubs, cafes, libraries, and museums – are often in touch with the traditionally 'hard-to-reach' groups.

35. National government, too, has a part to play. We are promoting better and safer local environments, access to cycle paths and the countryside, and decent housing through policies on local government, transport, law and order, and the environment. For many adults – including older people – an active lifestyle may not involve formal sport. We have already legislated through the Countryside Rights of Way Act to increase opportunities for active recreation in our countryside. Factors as simple as the attractiveness and perceived safety of the local environment are crucial if people are not to be pushed into an essentially sedentary lifestyle. And access to safe cycle paths, and to the countryside, will also promote public health. The recent *Review of the National Service Framework for Older People*[5] identifies action to improve the health and quality of life for older people in line with the principles of this White Paper.

4   *At Least Five a Week: evidence on the impact of physical activity and its relationship to health*, Chief Medical Officer, April 2004.
5   *Better Health in Old Age*, Report from Professor Ian Philp, National Director for Older People's Health to Secretary of State for Health: Department of Health, 2 November 2004.

CASE STUDY

"I am trying to bring my kids up to cycle. However, it is extremely hard. Cycling is fun, kids love it, it is environmentally friendly, quiet (ie no noisy engines) and very good exercise. Yet there is almost no opportunity to cycle. Where are the family-friendly cycle paths? How can a family cycle to the park? Or to school? To the shops? Or to visit friends?? There isn't an option to cycle. It isn't safe."

Mother

"I would rather 'pop-off' when I'm in the dance group than lie alone in my room waiting ... to die..." Rose's words encapsulated the ethos of the impact of an extraordinary 18-month National Lottery dance initiative for the elderly, based in three sheltered housing units and a residential home in Bristol. Many of the 80 and 90 year olds were relatively immobile and couldn't stand for long; yet all were challenged physically and imaginatively by performing in front of one another. The project brought out the youthful spirit of the elderly and encouraged social contact.

Ruth Sidgwick, project coordinator for Burn and Rave, believes implicitly that group members, "became ambassadors for the work" by speaking about themselves and their dance experiences in public places, such as conferences, as well as for their peers. One particular group was very keen to go into a local school to share with the pupils what they learnt.

36. We are committed to leading the delivery of cleaner, safer, greener public spaces and improvement of the quality of the built environment in deprived areas and across the country, with a national target to achieve measurable improvement by 2008. The Department of Culture Media and Sport will set out in more detail the Government's strategic approach to sport and physical activity in its five-year plan, to be published shortly.

37. The *Cleaner, Safer, Greener Communities* programme, led by the Office of the Deputy Prime Minister, addresses the relationship between the quality of the local environment and the quality of life. Individuals are obviously not capable of providing this quality of local environment on their own. They need the collective action of local government and community action. Higher-quality environments lead to greater use of public spaces and increase opportunities for people to choose healthy lifestyles. The programme priorities, to which local authorities are central, include creating attractive parks and open spaces, improving the physical fabric, making public places cleaner and maintaining them better, making places safer, providing for children and young people, tackling inequalities and engaging and empowering local communities.

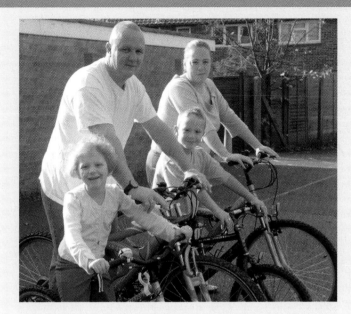

The Liveability Fund, announced as part of the Sustainable Communities Plan in 2003, is testing a new approach to addressing public space issues and focuses on improving local authorities' arrangements for managing and maintaining public space before investing in new developments. Twenty-seven local pilot areas were announced early this year and lessons and good practice will be disseminated throughout the process. It aims to ensure that parks and public spaces will be better managed and maintained and physical improvements will be more sustainable.

38. We will use lessons learned from the 27 local authority pilots on improving parks and public places in the development of the £660 million Safer and Stronger Communities Fund announced in Spending Review 2004.

39. Opportunities – provided by local authorities, and the voluntary and private sector – can play an important part in increasing physical activity, but it is also important to incorporate exercise into daily life. Walking and cycling present practical, alternative forms of activity that can be part of the daily routine for most people. The Government and its partners have already begun to create a better environment to walk or cycle. Under Department for Transport guidance, local authority investment in cycling facilities has increased by more than 30%:

- **The transport charity Sustrans, in partnership with local authorities, has already completed 8,000 miles of new cycle lanes and tracks, and local authorities are forecast to build over 7,000 miles of new cycle lanes and cycle tracks by 2006.**
- **The Department for Transport is investing in programmes to link the existing *National Cycle Network* to hundreds of schools, enabling more children to walk or cycle to school. This complements the wider *Travelling to School* programme.**
- **We will also be incorporating local highways authorities' statutory plans for improving public rights of way into local transport plans.**

40. Following evaluation, we will build on the *Sustainable Travel Towns* pilots to develop guidance for local authorities, PCTs and others on whole-town approaches to shifting travel from cars to walking, cycling and public transport. Locally, public health professionals in PCTs and Government Offices for the Regions will have a key role in leading development of local travel plans.

41. But even with this improved environment for walkers and cyclists, there are behavioural and

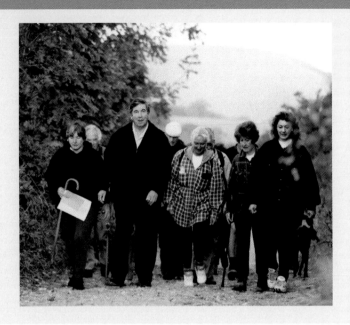

psychological barriers to overcome. People need to see the benefits of not taking the easy option of hopping into the car for short trips. Improving information on the opportunities to walk and cycle will be part of the strategy for marketing health set out in Chapter 2. Chapter 5 sets out the action we are taking to provide personal support for people in improving their health. NHS-accredited health trainers will provide a new resource for people to get individual advice and help in putting their ambitions to do more physical exercise into practice.

42. SkillsActive, the Sector Skills Council for active learning and leisure, will work alongside Skills for Health to enhance the skills of exercise professionals, coaches and others within the SkillsActive workforce. This is to ensure that they are able to fulfil health trainer roles and to establish a core set of skills and knowledge across sectors. In addition, health specialists will be able to undertake accreditation, to enable them to work in recreational activity settings.

Pedometers

Last summer, the Department of Health, working with the Countryside Agency and DEFRA, piloted the use of pedometers (or step-o-meters) in the NHS across 120 PCTs. The evaluation concluded that pedometers distributed by health professionals were a useful motivational tool in adults to encourage more walking (on average 1,600 extra steps a day). The pilot also found that awareness of the importance of exercise to both staff and patients in PCTs increased. An earlier pilot found that general postal distribution of pedometers (ie giving one to anyone who applies) is not effective; 42% of those who had requested a pedometer did not actually use it.

43. Motivation can matter as much as opportunity. Evidence from pilots suggests that wearing a pedometer can encourage people to walk more, especially when linked with wider programmes of activity. Given the increasing popularity of pedometers being offered commercially either for sale or as part of food marketing programmes or public information campaigns in the national media, **we will, as part of our proposals on marketing health outlined in Chapter 2, commission practical guidance on how to meet the Chief Medical Officer's physical activity recommendations, including the use of pedometers.**

CASE STUDY

The Walking the Way to Health initiative, launched by the British Heart Foundation and the Countryside Agency, is on track to get more than one million people walking more, to reduce their risk of coronary heart disease, stroke, diabetes, osteoporosis and obesity. The aim is to reach those who do not consider themselves 'walkers', including those who live in areas of 'poor health'. Trained volunteers plan and lead walks for those who like walking in company. Health walk routes are selected and promoted to people who prefer to walk independently. Doctors are also encouraging their patients to walk more.

Four years into its five-year life, around 900,000 people are walking more to benefit their health, 300 local communities have set up local schemes to promote 'walking for health' and 10,000 volunteers have been trained to lead walks.

44. **Working with the Countryside Agency, DEFRA and other partners, we will encourage health professionals across PCTs to use pedometers in clinical practice, with coverage of all areas by the end of 2005.**

45. **We are also working with the Youth Sports Trust to pilot the use of pedometers in schools – both as a tool to support a wide range of curriculum topics and to increase awareness amongst pupils of the need to be active.**

46. Other partners also have contributions to make. We are working with Sport England and the Countryside Agency on the *Local Exercise Action Pilot* programme to get people more active. The pilots have shown how successful partnerships between the NHS, local authorities, schools and community groups can be in encouraging adults and children to be more active. **Building on the success of the *Local Exercise Action* pilots, we will invest over the next three years in initiatives to promote physical activity supported by guidance to promote best practice. This will include:**

- **a Physical Activity Promotion Fund to roll out evidence-based physical activity interventions – linked where appropriate to local health trainers and developing obesity care services (see Chapter 6);**

- **regional Physical Activity Coordinators to coordinate delivery of activity interventions and support planning for use of the Fund, linked to plans to tackle obesity;**
- **guidance on what works for local authorities, PCTs and voluntary bodies, backed up by annual stakeholder events to promote best practice.**

SPORT'S UNIQUE CONTRIBUTION

47. Sport and active recreation make a significant contribution towards overall physical activity levels in the population – more than 30% of people took part in some form of active recreation at least once a week during 2002. Today's busy lifestyles and the availability of a wider range of sedentary pursuits are increasingly creating competing pressures. Yet sport in the broadest sense, which includes everyday activity, is attractive to many and offers people the kind of social networks described at the start of the chapter. And there is evidence that the right kind of investment can generate very significant increases in participation.

CASE STUDY

Plymouth Primary Care Trust and Plymouth City Council are running a free swimming programme for vulnerable and hard-to-reach young people in the city, as one of its Local Exercise Action Pilots. This aims to increase levels of physical activity and sports participation. Free swimming access, youth clubs in water, lifesaving, inflatable fun sessions, and diving and swimming lessons are being offered to 1,000 13–14 year olds from across the city over a two-year period. Young people are nominated for the scheme using a multi-agency referral process working in collaboration with schools and health, youth and community professionals.

48. Sport England's Framework for Sport, published in 2004, sets out the strategic direction for sport in England and their commitment to increasing opportunities for participation through the nine Regional Plans for Sport. In the regions, the Big Lottery Fund and Sport England are together investing £108 million in community sport and physical activity initiatives to engage new partners and participants with a special focus on areas of multiple deprivation.

49. The Government is backing the bid for London to stage the 2012 Olympic and Paralympic Games. The bid provides an opportunity to demonstrate the importance of sport and physical activity to improving health. The preparation for and, if successful, staging of the Games will provide the means for increasing public awareness of how to get more active. It will also be an opportunity to increase the usage of existing and new facilities built for the Games across our communities. **The Government, working with the NHS, British Olympic Association, Greater London Authority and London 2012 Ltd, will make clear the beneficial effects for Londoners, and the rest of the country, of increased physical activity.**

50. A number of local authorities have piloted free-swimming or wider free sports opportunities during school holidays. Some have also run schemes for pensioners during quieter periods in the pool.

We will work with key interests to develop best practice guidance on providing free swimming and other sport initiatives, for publication in 2005.

51. Football and other sports have a huge reach and engagement, and a strong community base. The Government is working with football and other sports to build on the many successful partnerships for health that already exist between professional football clubs and their local PCT and local authority. These include both opportunities for physical activity and wider action to communicate healthy lifestyle messages. As a next step, **we will publish a guide for PCTs and sports clubs to encourage good practice and foster links on health improvement work, building on existing work with football clubs and extending this to other sports.**

PROMOTING HEALTH AND SPORT MEDICINE

52. We recognise, of course, that one of the consequences of encouraging people to be more active is that people may sustain more injuries and will also need expert advice on promoting their health through activity. We are currently consulting the medical profession on the recognition of sport and exercise medicine as a specialty within the NHS. Subject to the consultation responses, this should lead to the training and placement within the NHS of more doctors who will have a positive

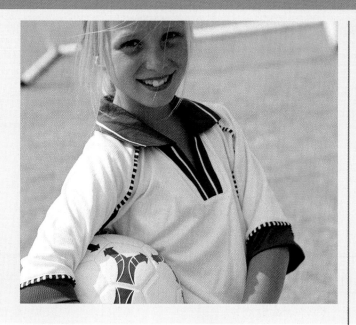

CASE STUDY

role in promoting health and are specifically trained to deal with such injuries and to give advice on how to exercise safely to stop such injuries recurring in future.

WIDER OPPORTUNITIES FOR IMPROVING HEALTH
Prevention of accidents

53. Local action is also important in preventing accidents in the home and on the streets. We will commission the Royal Society for the Prevention of Accidents to establish an accreditation scheme for safety centres across England to sustain best practice and new ways of delivering accident-prevention messages.

CORPORATE SOCIAL RESPONSIBILITY FOR HEALTH

54. Many local and national employers, businesses and voluntary bodies are already beginning to respond to people's wish for better health.

55. Corporate social responsibility (CSR) driven by values and applied consistently across a company's activities can be a powerful tool for good. Companies have the opportunity to improve the environment in which individuals make their healthy choices. They can achieve changes that individuals on their own cannot.

Positive Futures is a social inclusion programme which uses sport to reduce anti-social behaviour and drug misuse. On St Mary's estate in Bargate, Southampton, ranked the 49th most deprived ward in England and Wales, the Positive Futures coordinator has run football sessions for the most disengaged 13 to 16 year olds, many of whom are referred to the project by schools, social services, local police and the youth service.

Gradually, through getting to know the young people on the football pitch, the coordinator builds up some trust and encourages the teenagers to visit the project's youth club, which takes place three nights a week. Eventually, some are even willing to attend a study club, and get involved in homework groups and learning IT skills. A weekly multi-sport session has been held for 10 to 12 year olds at the local leisure centre, where they can try a variety of sports, free from bullying by older teenagers. Five young people previously connected to the project have already started a BTEC course in Sport and Leisure at Totton College.

'It is possible for the NHS to become an organisation that promotes health and sustainable development, thereby increasing its own chances of a sustainable future. For that to happen, however, incentives will have to be geared to encourage and reward changes in corporate behaviour.'

Claiming the Health Dividend: unlocking the benefits of NHS spending, King's Fund report

Building engagement through champions for health

56. In responses to *Choosing Health?* many organisations told us what they were already doing to improve health, and others made new commitments to action. We want to build on this.

57. The Improvement and Development Agency for local government (IDeA) has pledged to work with the NHS Modernisation Agency to encourage the growth of local leadership skills for health. This will include development of networks of people who will support action to improve people's health in local communities. **We will work with others to develop a network of health champions, starting in local government but drawing from a wide range of organisations and sectors – including voluntary organisations and individuals who want to champion health. Nationally, we will support local health champions through arrangements to share good practice and celebrate success through an annual award scheme that recognises excellence and commitment to improve health.** Health champions will be people with experience, enthusiasm and often skills in promoting health and community engagement. These champions will be able to offer short-term consultancy support to local councils and community partnerships to share good practice and assist them in developing local action for health.

58. Following on from the interest shown in the *Choosing Health?* consultation we will invite national and local organisations to make their own pledges about what they will do to respond to people's enthusiasm to improve their health. This may be a pledge to their own workforce, to their local community, to their customers, or form part of their core business.

59. Organisations will be invited to communicate their pledge in their own way. But we shall also invite them to record their pledge publicly, as part of the response to the public interest in seeing action on health. We propose establishing a website hosted from outside government, on which organisations may post pledges and members of the public respond. We will celebrate what organisations and individual health champions achieve through an annual award system that recognises excellence and commitment to improve people's health.

Corporate social responsibility for health in the NHS

60. Just as we are seeking greater leadership in corporate social responsibility from the private sector, the NHS must play a similar role for the public sector. The NHS operates as the biggest business in England and will be spending £90 billion by 2008. As the country's largest employer and with a total spend on food, goods and services which represents some 10% of regional economies, NHS

CASE STUDY

organisations can and must make a significant contribution to the health and sustainability of the communities they serve.

61. Many NHS organisations have already recognised their impact on health, the local economy and the environment. Increasingly, rapid growth in the NHS is supporting people from disadvantaged areas and groups by creating jobs in NHS organisations and developing the skills of local people. In deprived areas, the NHS is often the biggest local employer, helping to improve the prosperity of communities with relatively high levels of worklessness and health inequalities.

62. With rising levels of investment, as the NHS continues to grow to meet the needs of local communities, it is increasing demand for goods and services. That demand is increasingly being met by local suppliers, and local social enterprise is being expanded. Capital developments, including hospital building programmes and Local Improvement Finance Trust (LIFT), are providing local jobs, helping people develop new skills, and creating new business opportunities to meet the needs of an expanding NHS. They also act as a catalyst for local community engagement in health and provide opportunities to ensure that developments are sustainable. This is benefiting individuals and their families, and contributing to local economies and to community wellbeing.

Doorstep Greens is a £20 million initiative, which is helping up to 200 communities in urban and rural England to create greens that are safe, enjoyable to use and meet the needs of local residents. Managed by the Countryside Agency with funding from the Big Lottery Fund, it aims to improve access and use of local green space, especially in socially and economically disadvantaged areas, as communities are encouraged to plan, design, create and manage their own green space.

The AMC Gardens in a deprived area of Nottingham is one example which began as a derelict piece of ground which is now transformed into a garden, part of which is given over to growing vegetables for local use. In Witham in Essex, the local community have taken on the management of a run-down park and turned it into an enjoyable place for children to play and exercise.

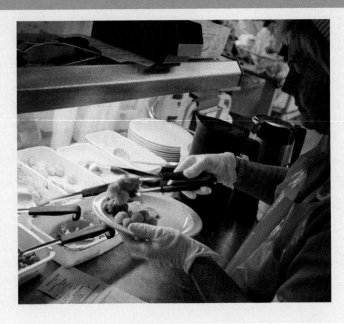

63. We need to do much more if we are to realise the full potential of the NHS. The NHS Chief Executive, Sir Nigel Crisp, has identified the role of the NHS as a good corporate citizen as one of his five new priorities for the next ten years. As part of that work, **we will fund the Sustainable Development Commission's *Healthy Futures* programme to develop the capacity of NHS organisations to act as good corporate citizens. This will include the development of a self-assessment model to help assess progress. We will develop guidance on good practice in:**

- **food procurement in the NHS and across other public sector services;[6] and**
- **capital developments and new building programmes in the NHS.[7]**

64. Catering providers in both the public and private sector have an important role to play in influencing access to healthier foods. Public procurement of food through the NHS, the Prison Service and the Ministry of Defence offers an opportunity to demonstrate best practice. **We will develop nutritional standards for all foods provided by these organisations and other public bodies – building on the work in schools. Our intention is to increase access to a range of healthier foods and will take account of the different formats of food provision – restaurant, fast food, vending, etc.** This will be supported by

a new Working Group and will link into the work of the Public Sector Food Procurement Initiative led by DEFRA and the work of the Expert Panel on Armed Forces Feeding (EPAFF), recently set up by the Ministry of Defence. We will look at opportunities to promote this guidance into the private sector through the introduction of a national 'Healthy Eating' award. This will build on local initiatives, often promoted by environmental health, such as 'Heartbeat' awards.

65. In developing its own corporate citizenship programme, the NHS will seek to draw on good practice wherever it exists. **The Government will sponsor debate on corporate citizenship across the public sector that leads to firm recommendations for action for all public and private sector employers, to demonstrate how they can organise their activities in ways that improve the health of employees and the wider community.** The goal will be to establish a set of standards that can be adopted by a wide range of organisations over time.

66. The problems connected with poor accessibility of services, including health services, represent huge costs for individuals, communities and the state. It is particularly problematic as it makes it difficult for people to access health care services and has implications for the NHS in seeking to achieve its targets. The Social Exclusion Unit's 2003 report *Making the Connections* showed that

---

6 Linking in to the work of the new Regional Centres of Excellence for the local government sector and other public sector services and linked to the work outlined earlier in this chapter.

7 Capital developments, including LIFT, within the NHS should be able to demonstrate their consideration to sustainability and build this into their capital build processes. Through the Building for Health programme in London, a model of how to do this and an approach and toolkit to support trusts has been developed with trusts and PFI developers. www.nhsestates.gov.uk/sustainable_development/content/neat.html

CASE STUDY

City and Hackney Teaching Primary Care Trust offers a generous travel allowance to cyclists of 34p per mile. The bicycle users group proposed, and have now implemented, a bicycle pool scheme. With a grant from the Primary Care Trust's Health Improvement Directorate, the group purchased bikes, together with safety equipment and maintenance kit. All staff can register to use the bikes, free of charge, for work purposes and have the opportunity to register for free cycling lessons.

during the course of a year 1.4 million people will miss, turn down or not even seek hospital appointments because of problems with transport and that 31% of those without a car have difficulties travelling to their local hospital, compared to 17% with a car.

67. Accessibility Planning can make a significant contribution to the achievement of the Department of Health aim to 'transform the health and social care system so that it produces faster, fairer services that deliver better health and tackle health inequalities'. We will encourage NHS bodies to work with local authorities as they draw up accessibility plans by July 2005 to improve access to health services.

68. NHS organisations will need to work in partnership with others. Regional Development Agencies have recognised the potential benefit from working with the NHS to achieve health and economic development objectives. Working locally to support employment and skills development strategies, and participating in planning activity for sustainable development, local transport and the environment will enable PCTs and NHS trusts to ensure a positive impact on the health of local people. Involvement will also enable NHS organisations to shape long-term plans for investment in new property, to meet the needs of changing local populations.

NHS staff, patients and visitors in England and Wales travelled an estimated 25 billion passenger kilometres in 2001. Of these, 21 billion (81%) passenger kilometres were travelled by car and van.

Source: Material Health

SMOKE-FREE PUBLIC PLACES

69. Exposure to second-hand smoke is one topic where nationally and locally individuals and communities have already generated pressure for action to improve health choices. This is one of the most hotly debated issues, involving as it does a conflict between individual rights, and between rights and responsibilities in society.

70. Three-quarters of respondents in the Opinion Leader Research (OLR) survey agreed that the Government should prevent people from doing things that put the health of others at risk. People want to see a shift in the balance between the rights of the minority of people who choose to smoke and the rights of other people whose health or enjoyment may be adversely affected by second-hand smoke. They do not, however, believe that this requires a complete ban in all licensed premises.

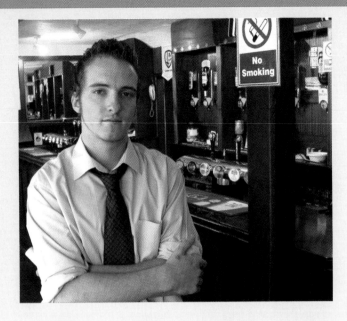

71. The evidence of risk to health from exposure to second-hand smoke points towards an excess number of deaths, although debate on the precise scale of the impact continues. The consultation demonstrated clear concerns about both the health impact and discomfort felt by many in smoke-filled environments, with particular concerns about locations such as work places, where people may not have been able to choose to be in a smoke-free environment.

72. As the stark new warnings on cigarette packs say 'Smoking seriously harms you and others around you'. Among the conditions linked to second-hand smoke are:

- lung cancer;
- heart disease;
- asthma attacks; and
- sudden infant death syndrome.

73. The best way that smokers can reduce the risk to themselves of those diseases that are caused by smoking is by giving up. That is why Chapters 5 and 6 put such emphasis on providing information and support to help individuals give up. But as a society we can act to help smokers to make that difficult healthy choice and stick to it. We know that one of the greatest benefits from smoke-free public places is that people trying to give up

smoking can find it easier to succeed if social pressures not to smoke are increased.

74. There has already been significant response across society. Thirty years ago, 46% of people in England smoked. Today it is 26%. By 2003, some 50% of people said their workplace was completely smoke-free, and in total 88% of people said their workplace had some form of smoking restriction in place. But the evidence from the consultation and from public surveys is that this is not enough. Repeatedly, the message from the large majority of smokers as well as non-smokers is that one of the ways to improve their local opportunities for health is through smoke-free settings.

75. Some workplaces are also primarily places where people come together to drink alcohol. Views about the case for smoking bans in pubs were different from views on workplaces as a whole. Surveys and opinion polls consistently show some 86% of people in favour of workplace restrictions, and a similarly substantial majority of people supporting restrictions in restaurants. But when people are asked whether smoking should be restricted in pubs the figures fall substantially – to around 56% – and when people are asked which sort of restrictions they would prefer in pubs only 20% of people choose 'no smoking allowed

anywhere' and the majority tend to be opposed to a complete ban.

76. Nevertheless, this is an area where people cannot readily secure change for themselves. In our 1998 White Paper *Smoking Kills* we were clear that fast and substantial progress was needed: we decided that the case for legal action to restrict smoking was not, at that time, sufficiently strong. However, change has been slow and public demand for action has increased. It is one of the few instances in this White Paper where we believe the right response is Government action in the form of legislation.

We therefore intend to shift the balance significantly in favour of smoke-free environments. Subject to parliamentary timetables, we propose to regulate, with legislation where necessary, in order to ensure that:

- **all enclosed public places and workplaces (other than licensed premises which are dealt with below) will be smoke-free;**
- **licensed premises will be treated as follows:**
  - **all restaurants will be smoke-free;**
  - **all pubs and bars preparing and serving food will be smoke-free;**
  - **other pubs and bars will be free to choose whether to allow smoking or to be smoke-free;**
  - **in membership clubs the members will be free to choose whether to allow smoking or to be smoke-free; and**
  - **smoking in the bar area will be prohibited everywhere.**

77. We intend to introduce smoke-free places through a staged approach:

- **by the end of 2006, all government departments and the NHS will be smoke-free;**
- **by the end of 2007, all enclosed public places and workplaces, other than licensed premises (and those specifically exempted), will, subject to legislation, be smoke-free;**
- **by the end of 2008 arrangements for licensed premises will be in place.**

We will use the intervening period of time to consult widely in the process of drawing up the detailed legislation, including on the special arrangements needed for regulating smoking in certain establishments – such as hospices, prisons and long stay residential care. In implementing this policy there are also a range of practical issues that will need to be addressed – we will need to consult, for example, with schools and other institutions on how best to give practical effect to this policy, as well as how best to enforce the policy and what penalties will be appropriate for people who do not follow the law.

Some have pointed to a risk inherent in this proposal that pubs may decide to stop serving food instead of imposing a smoking ban; and that this may have an adverse impact on our drive to tackle binge-drinking. We believe that the profitability of providing food will be sufficient to outweigh any perverse incentive for pub owners to choose to switch. However, we will consult widely with all those engaged in combating irresponsible drinking to ensure the risk is mitigated, and will monitor outcomes.

78. We believe these measures respond to what we have heard, striking the right balance between responsibilities and freedoms. They will represent a major advance, making smoke-free public places the norm.

79. Based on the current make-up of pubs we estimate that 10 to 30% might fall into the category of 'do not prepare food' – meaning around 10 to 30% of pubs could be smoking, and the remainder smoke-free.

CONCLUSION

80. We have learnt much over the past few years about how new forms of community action and leadership can make a real difference to people's lives. These examples have demonstrated how people together can achieve more than individuals alone. We need to unleash this potential for health, starting with the roll out of models driven by communities for health. Government will act to hasten progress towards a smoke-free public environment and – in partnership with others – to increase opportunities for activity. The public sector, led by local authorities with PCTs, will need to play its part. Independent sector organisations, nationally and locally, are already demonstrating their commitment.

Delivery Task Group's top three messages to Community Groups:

- don't accept poor health as inevitable – promote the message that people can change their circumstances;
- help people in your communities to feel more in control of their lives – if you can affect the neighbourhood you live in, people may begin to believe they can affect their own life chances;
- look for small achievements – examples of things that your community can do to improve health – and shout about your successes.

81. In doing so we will strengthen the health, social and economic infrastructure of local communities and provide supportive environments for making healthy choices. This will be supported through wider action to develop local ties, improve community cohesion, local prosperity and local environments, and to reduce inequalities, crime and social exclusion. None of these problems is easy to tackle and change will take time, commitment, energy, resources, and strong local leadership to promote effective partnerships.

82. The drive to face up to these challenges can only come through engagement with the reality of people's lives in the communities they live in. Government investment and public sector reform is playing its part in helping to develop the basic support and improvement to facilitate such change, and future Government programmes will continue to support and enhance this effort.

The commitments in this chapter will mean that:

- successful community-based models for improving local health can be more confident of sustained support;
- local authorities and PCTs will have more flexibility to develop local targets through local partnership, in response to local needs;
- there will be new opportunities for people who want to be more active through cycling, walking, and easier access to sports facilities;
- organisations, including NHS organisations, will increasingly use their corporate power in ways that promote the health and wellbeing of their local communities;
- people across all sectors of society will be encouraged to work together to improve health; and
- there will be new opportunities for people to work and socialise in places that are smoke-free.

5 Health as a way of life

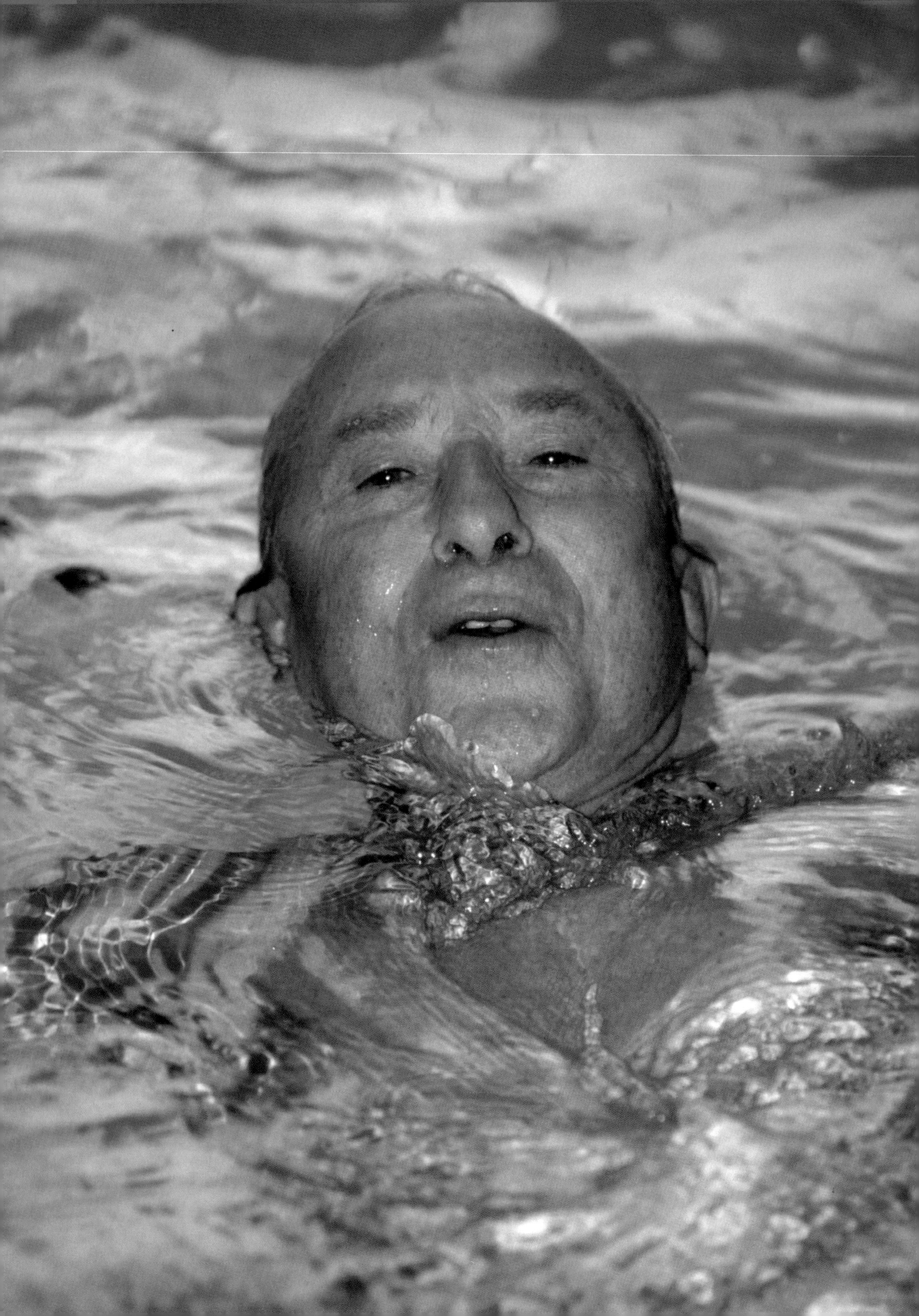

CHAPTER SUMMARY

The consultation made it clear that people are ambitious for their health and the health of their families, but often found it difficult to turn good intentions into sustained action. People wanted support both in making the right decisions for their own health and help to carry them out in practice. This chapter sets out new proposals to provide that support.

- *First, anyone who wants help to make healthier choices and stick to them will have the opportunity to be supported by a new kind of personal health resource, NHS health trainers. In keeping with a shift in public health approaches from 'advice from on high to support from next door', health trainers will be drawn from local communities, understanding the day-to-day concerns and experiences of the people they are supporting on health. They will be accredited by the NHS to have skills appropriate for helping members of their community to achieve the changes that they want to make. In touch with the realities of the lives of the people they work with and with a shared stake in improving the health of the communities that they live in, health trainers will be friendly, approachable, understanding and supportive. Offering practical advice and good connections into the services and support available locally, they will become an essential common-sense resource in the community to help out on health choices. A guide for those who want help, not an instructor for those who do not, they will provide valuable support for people to make informed lifestyle choices. Different neighbourhoods will need different types of health trainers and in developing good practice we will learn from seeing which models work best for different communities and individuals. By starting in the most deprived communities we will learn how best to ensure that health trainers reach the most deprived groups.*

- *Second, everyone who wants to will have the opportunity, starting in the areas of the country with the biggest health challenges, to use a personal health kit to develop their own personal health plan, based on who **they** are, what **they** want and what **their** circumstances are. This tool will help people to identify their own priorities for health, the changes that they feel ready to make, to receive online guidance about what will make the most impact to their lives and receive tailored advice on how to go about making changes and sticking to them.*

"It is so reassuring to have someone to help you when you are not sure and have someone to help you going through things like when your children are ready for their injections. The learning material is simpler to understand than other health information available."

"When I first got pregnant, I knew I had to cut down on coffee and alcohol and finally face up to the fact that I really should be eating five fruit and vegetables a day; my body told me I needed more water. I tried to read as much as possible about healthy eating habits for pregnant women. There's a lot of advice out there but it's knowing where to go and who to ask."

Mother

INTRODUCTION

1. Millions of people are trying to lose weight. Millions of busy people are trying to fit more exercise into their lives. 70% of England's 10 million smokers want to stop smoking. Millions of parents are looking for cheap and convenient ways to provide good food for their children. That strong desire by millions of individuals in England to change to a healthier way of life is an opportunity.

2. The difficulty people experience in changing to a healthier way of life is a call for action. As most of us know, turning intention into sustained change is not easy. Too often an unsuccessful attempt on our own to change deep-seated habits leads to feelings of failure, even guilt, and a frustrating lack of control over our lives. For many people, although they often understand the harm involved in not changing their ways, the apparently insurmountable problems in doing so lead them to think that healthy choices are simply not for them. Lectures from distant national bodies and worthy exhortation to change from well-intentioned organisations with seemingly weak connections to the realities of everyday life can become irritating reminders of these negative feelings about health. As a result, too often good intentions are put in a 'too difficult' box and not followed through.

3. The nature of public health action itself must change if we are to break this cycle. Initiatives to increase demand for healthy choices need to be matched, when people want it, with support that fits with individual needs on the ground. Health policies and actions must change if we are to make a positive impact on people's health. Individuals look to Government for practical help by making the environment more conducive to healthy choices. Individuals cannot change their whole environment on their own.

4. Earlier chapters have already described how we will seek to create a consumer environment that makes change easier; to help build communities that support healthier choices; and make a concerted effort to prevent the development of unhealthy behaviours in childhood. But people also need to have greater power over their own health. This chapter sets out the support that will be made available to individuals, so that when they do want to act, and want help in doing so, they are not left on their own.

5. There is already some support. But it is patchy, fragmented and often does not fit with the realities of everyday lives. It might be on offer but at the wrong time when people are at work or have to look after their children. It might be only available to people who speak English well. Access is unequal and erratic. As a result, for too many, the healthy choice is still the most difficult option and

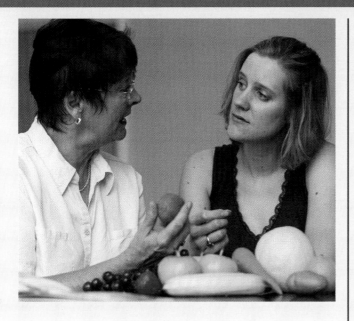

CASE STUDY

those most in need of help often get the least support, making inequalities in health worse.

6. This chapter sets out action to provide people who would like help in adopting a healthier way of life with practical support from people who understand the sorts of pressures and problems they face. It also sets out some tools that people can use, if they want, to make their own guides for health and to think through how best to put them into practice.

7. In doing so it seeks to put in place an infrastructure that is able to reach out to people in particularly difficult circumstances and provide them with relevant practical support. Success will be critical to tackling inequalities in health. It will mean building on approaches that are proven to be effective with people who are often left out of mainstream action on health or who have lost confidence in their ability to improve their health. It also means using the local economic power of the NHS as a source for regeneration in local communities by providing local jobs for local people.

PERSONAL SUPPORT
8. People often need practical support to turn their hopes for their own health into action – and to stick at it. Some of this help may already be available in local communities, with slimmers' clubs, groups who plan walks or other physical activities, food co-ops,

Voluntary sector organisation Age Concern, in partnership with local health organisations in an inner London borough, adopted a community development approach to encourage middle-aged men and women living in a multicultural area to develop personalised health plans. They initially lobbied local leisure facilities to provide services which more accurately met the needs and aspirations of people in midlife.

The support service was offered at a range of community venues such as healthy living centres, faith premises and community halls. A health check with a healthcare professional at the local GP surgery was provided as an optional follow-on service along with support from a community development worker to implement the personalised health plan. The formation of a focus group proved worthwhile as group encouragement from their peers supported individuals to make the lifestyle changes necessary to improve their health. A video was even produced which discussed different women's experiences of middle age living in Hackney.

One user commented, "My mental health is much better, which has helped my physical health because now instead of saying I'm too tired to go out, I'll say right, I'm going to go out and I'm going to meet so and so."

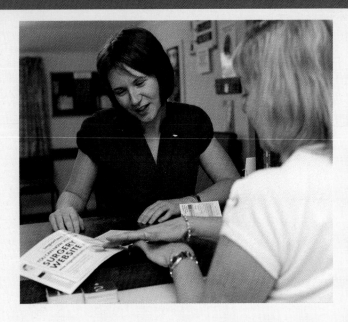

or groups for new mothers. The problem is that access to this sort of facility is too often a matter of chance or down to the efforts of a few committed individuals, rather than the result of a systematic approach to ensure comprehensive access to support on improving health.

9. People get advice and support from a very wide range of sources – families, friends, the media and their local community. In future, to supplement this, everyone who wants to will also be able to access personalised advice from health trainers, properly and professionally trained, and accredited by the NHS.

10. From 2006, NHS-accredited health trainers will be giving support to people who want it in the areas with highest need[1] and from 2007 progressively across the country. The new services will be developed first in deprived communities, and we will take account of emerging experience and best practice as the service is developed in other areas. Primary Care Trusts (PCTs) and children's trusts, working together with community organisations, health professionals and local authorities, will agree how best to provide this support to reach even the most deprived groups.

11. In keeping with a shift in public health approaches from 'advice from on high to support from next door', health trainers will often come from local communities. They will be accredited by the NHS to have proven skills to help local people make the changes that they want to. Health trainers will be friendly, approachable, understanding and supportive. It is sometimes hard to change the habits of a lifetime without some support. They will be people who are in touch with the realities of the lives of the people with whom they work and connected through a shared stake in improving the health of the communities that they live in.

12. Offering practical support instead of preaching, and good connections into the advice and support available locally, they will become an essential practical resource in the community to 'help out' on health choices – a guide for those who want help, not an instructor for those who do not. Different neighbourhoods will need different types of health trainers and in developing good practice we will learn from seeing which models work best for different communities and individuals.

13. In some communities people from a variety of organisations and walks of life are already performing a similar role and the evidence is that they can have a real impact. While there will be a core set of skills that every health trainer will need to receive accreditation, local models will need to build on the skills and strengths of the people who are already working in these kinds of role.

1   Those 20% of PCTs with the worst health and deprivation indicators.

CASE STUDY

Fahmeda, and another health promotion specialist, have been involved in organising various health improvement activities with South Asian groups in Middlesbrough, including a health event at the Hindu Cultural Centre. This promoted healthy eating, smoking cessation and taking measurements of height and weight. A diabetes nurse attended and wider issues such as housing were also addressed. Leaflets on various health topics were translated into Hindi and distributed. Feedback from the event indicates that the service was a great success and the community has asked for it to be repeated.

Fahmeda has also worked together with colleagues at the PCT to run a pilot weight management and coronary heart disease awareness programme with Asian women over 50. She visits the Sahara women's community group, who meet on a weekly basis, to check their weight and give basic advice on diet, for example reducing salt intake and cutting down on fat by using cooking oil rather than ghee. Fahmeda also suggests ways that the women can introduce more physical activity into their lifestyle such as through housework and walking.

14. Providing information and persuasive messages can increase people's knowledge of health risks and what action to take to deal with them. This is an essential framework for changing our way of life, but it is rarely enough on its own. There is good evidence that a range of approaches grounded in psychological science can help people in changing habits and behaviours. These sorts of approaches help people:

- learn how to watch for things around them that can trigger or reinforce the behaviour they want to change;
- set goals and plan how to achieve them; and
- build confidence to make the changes that they want to.

These important skills and techniques in supporting behavioural change will be a key element of health trainers' work as they have already proved to be effective in reaching out to people who are seeking help. Health trainers will need the skills and credibility to reach out and support people who need help most and find healthy choices harder to make, tailoring their work to individual's circumstances, recognising the problems people face and helping equip them with the skills and motivation to change.

15. In the past, many sources of advice have been designed around a single issue – help with giving

CASE STUDY

More than 500 adults have received health checks, and in excess of 1,000 children have completed healthy lifestyle workshops, at schools and community centres across Lincoln following the introduction in March 2003 of an initiative designed to increase physical activity.

The Community Health Assessment Programme (CHAP), which runs 14 different venues across Lincoln, offers adults free health checks measuring weight, blood pressure, heart rate, body fat, grip strength, body mass index and lung function. The one-to-one appointments are proving a success, with users' feedback praising the support given and claiming their health has improved as a result. Participants can attend as many times as they like to keep track of their levels and see how their lifestyle changes are making a difference.

Healthy lifestyle workshops, also part of the Lincoln City Initiative, offer a one-off session or six-week programme in which health issues are explored, including physical activities and warming up and cooling down. Children are given a workbook to go through with puzzles and colouring activities, and each participant is given a certificate and a goody bag when they reach the end of the programme.

Health and Fitness Development Officer, Jo Smith, said, "Most of the people we see are inactive and could really benefit from making some changes. For some of them, just suggesting simple lifestyle changes, like getting off a bus a stop earlier, is helpful whereas others would like to get more involved in more walks and what's going on in the city."

up smoking or losing weight, for example – rather than tackling life in the round. We want to make sure that people can start by accessing advice appropriate to them from one person who recognises their needs and motivations as an individual, not just as a smoker or a person who is overweight.

16. Individuals will be able to contact their health trainer through their local health centre, walk-in centre or by contacting NHS Direct. But health trainers will have a range of bases in the community and might also be employed by voluntary or community groups. Different neighbourhoods will have different needs, and we will learn from what works best.

17. People working in the NHS and other agencies such as social services, housing departments, or in the voluntary sector will be able to put people in touch with a health trainer if they think they would benefit from help with a change in lifestyle, or advice on coping with a temporary crisis or longer-term change in circumstances.

18. **If people want it, NHS-accredited health trainers will provide advice and support to develop a personal health guide, including help with:**

- **defining the changes they want to make;**

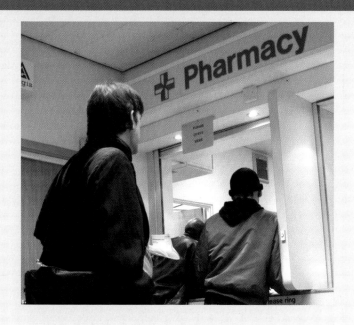

■ providing advice and practical support on what they can do – such as stopping smoking, doing more exercise, healthy eating, practising safe sex, dealing with stress or tackling social isolation;

■ providing advice, motivation and support – including training to look after their own health, advice, and help with making better use of lifestyle information – on making and sustaining changes over time; and

■ explaining how to access other help locally, both from the NHS and more widely across the community.

19. Health trainers will be able to offer people a health 'stock-take', to help them assess how their way of life might be impacting on their health and the sorts of changes that might be beneficial to them. This can be an effective way of preventing further inequalities in health through, for example, identifying people who may be at risk of developing chronic diseases or supporting people with existing chronic conditions. This sort of approach has been shown to be effective in work with people in their 50s – an age at which people often begin to experience illnesses that can develop into chronic disease and a time when people's motivation to improve their own health increases. By equipping people with the skills to look after their own health and providing them with support when it is needed, local services and health trainers can make a real impact in helping people to live longer and healthier lives.

20. NHS health trainers will be the fundamental building blocks for health improvement in the NHS to provide much needed new capacity and approaches to tackling inequalities. They will be accredited to provide general advice on improving health and on specific issues such as stopping smoking or changing diet as well as skills to look after their own health. For many people this sort of support will be all that they want. But people are not all the same and some may need more specialised help. Health trainers will be able to help people access other support, both from their local community and from specialised services such as the NHS Stop Smoking Services or sexual health services, or advice and support on diet and exercise that are described in more detail in Chapter 6.

21. Some groups of people find it difficult to access services designed to meet the needs of the general population and extra efforts will be needed to ensure that everyone has the opportunity to benefit from the new support available through health trainers – for example, some disabled people will want extra support. **We will offer disabled people the option of taking up a health stock-take as trailed in *Building on the Best: Choice, Equity and Responsiveness in the NHS* and will shortly consult on proposals to do so.**

CASE STUDY

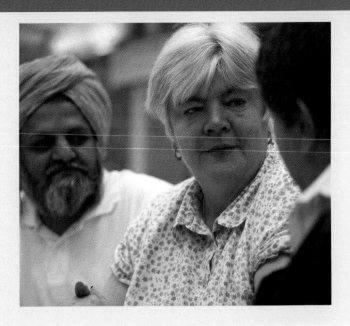

Sue Curtis, Head Dietician for Tameside and Glossop PCT, where she has worked for 16 years, is responsible for a number of award-winning, imaginative projects helping diabetic and overweight patients in the area to achieve a healthier lifestyle.

Obese patients can now participate at reduced cost in a range of dry land and water-based exercise activities thanks to a partnership she has built with Tameside Sports Trust Lifestyle Club, which runs at all six swimming pools and sports centres in the area.

Sue's team also developed the first Asian diabetes support worker team in the country to meet the particular needs of Asian patients and their families by training local people to become lifestyle course facilitators, leading free courses across the district helping people wishing to reduce their weight.

She also helped to set up the Tameside Healthy Choice Award Scheme, working with Tameside MBC Environmental Health Officers, to motivate a wide range of food businesses to improve their range of healthy food choices and reduce the range of less healthy ones. Virtually all secondary and primary schools in the area are now included in the scheme and are making significant improvements to obtain higher levels of award, graduating from bronze to silver and then gold.

22. Most health trainers will come from local communities and will work as part of NHS primary care services. The NHS, through PCTs, will take lead responsibility for ensuring that people in their area have access to such support and know how to use it.

23. The arrangements will differ according to the needs of a particular community. Just as each neighbourhood is different, each trainer will be different. In some areas health trainers may be people working in the NHS or voluntary sector who already fulfil a similar role in the community. In such cases, being a health trainer could be one element of their job role. In other areas, particularly those where there are marked health inequalities, it may be better to recruit and train new staff from the community as dedicated health trainers. This can also help provide new job opportunities for people in local communities.

Community matrons are ideally placed to promote the health of people with long-term conditions. In their hands-on, case management role they will identify those whose health is at greatest risk and work with the patient and their carers to reduce the effects of disease and prevent accidents, dehydration, infections or other conditions that could result in admission to hospital. Community matrons will also be able to put their patients in contact with NHS-accredited health trainers, who can provide additional practical support to the patient and carers on changing their behaviour to prevent further ill health.

24. NHS health trainers will need good training to fulfil this role. We will provide national core curriculum and training modules to ensure that skills are quality assured and standardised, and based on best practice principles of how to support lifestyle change.

25. There will be a competence framework for developing the necessary skills for health trainers. In order to ensure that a broad range of people become accredited, this framework will also be used to develop health improvement skills in existing workforces – including in the voluntary and sport and leisure sectors. Different sections of the training package will help a broad range of workers to develop specific health skills that could be used in their job, from equipping NHS staff to provide stop smoking advice or equipping community workers to provide general advice on health.

26. This new type of role will provide opportunities for local people to take the first step on a 'Skills Escalator' to improve and develop their skills through the National Qualifications Framework by developing skills for health improvement, prevention and behavioural change. It will extend opportunities to people currently providing advice and support in their local community who may not otherwise have considered a career in the NHS or the public sector. It will also increase opportunities for employment and development in the local community, enabling people to develop a role in providing advice to their community while developing their own understanding of health and community issues. The strategy extends opportunities for the NHS to use its economic power in the local community as a force for regeneration, creating jobs for local people that in turn support improvement in health across the communities they come from.

27. Health trainers will be just one element of a wider workforce geared for health improvement and prevention, ranging from those who provide patients with opportunistic advice on health

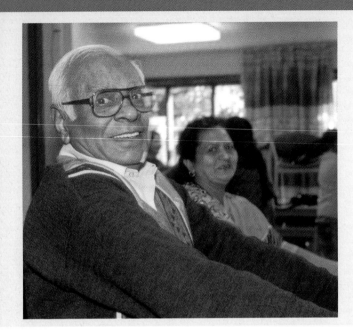

improvement in their day-to-day contacts to those whose job is dedicated to providing advice and support on health improvement. Health trainers will support colleagues in primary care with the additional skills in health improvement they bring to the workforce. Health trainers will be an integral part of a comprehensive local health improvement service and an NHS workforce that is properly and professionally geared up to promote health.

PLANNING FOR HEALTH

28. Many people want to work out their own plans to improve their health but would find it helpful to have a clear framework and the practical tools to get them started. We need to find ways of providing that help so that people, particularly in deprived areas and groups, can act on those aspirations.

29. Help and support needs to suit people's individual circumstances. Supporting a personal approach to health will help ensure that *everybody* has the opportunity to enjoy the best health they can. To make healthier choices, people need to want to be healthier, but when they come to that point, many feel that they also need help to set goals which they can achieve. Chapter 3 sets out action to help get children and young people on the right path. It can be equally important to provide help at other stages in life, when people take stock of where they have got to and where

they want to go next – before retirement, moving away from home for the first time, a special birthday, starting a family, or following the break up of a longstanding relationship.

30. In recent years there has been growing evidence of the success of the 'self-care' or 'expert patient' approaches to people when they are ill. This approach helps people to learn more about their own illness, and how to manage it effectively without always depending on professionals for support. It helps to put patients in control of their plans for how they manage their own disease. We need to extend this approach into prevention, before people develop illnesses, enabling people to take greater control of their own health and enabling them to plan for their health on their own terms.

31. **Starting from 2006 in the areas with highest need[2] and then progressively across the country by 2008, people, if they want to, will be able to use a variety of different types of support from the NHS to develop their own personal health guides.**

32. A personal health guide will be unique to every individual and give them the opportunity to:

- work out for themselves how healthy their current lifestyle is;
- set out their ambitions for their health; and

2   Those 20% of PCTs with the worst health and deprivation indicators.

SCENARIO
WHAT WILL HEALTH
LOOK LIKE IN THE
FUTURE?

Maggie is 55. She has never worked and lives alone with her son, who has severe learning disabilities. Luckily, she has never been ill herself but she occasionally feels a bit down and would like to do something that gets her out of the house once in a while – perhaps to take some exercise.

Her local PCT is worried about the isolation suffered by carers and works with a local voluntary group to create a portal site containing information about healthy lifestyles, benefits and support groups.

The site includes online discussion groups and a secure email service that carers can use to send queries to the PCT, social services and other agencies. Basic IT courses are organised at local community centres and colleges to deliver skills to carers and support their use of the site. Maggie arranges to do a two-hour course at her local library, which is a UK Online centre, while her son attends some day care. This gives her general information about how to log on to the internet, find and navigate the portal.

On the portal, she reads about a new health check being offered to people in their 50s. Maggie has always worried about how her son would cope if she were ill, so she decides to try the service.

Outreach clinics are also held at the library by the local health trainer. Maggie is encouraged to record her health record and family history. She discusses her health and concerns with the adviser who notes that, although she is a non-smoker and doesn't drink, she is overweight (BMI 27) and doesn't manage to eat five portions of fruit and vegetables a day or exercise for the recommended 30 minutes five days a week. She checks she has had cervical and breast screening tests, and offers to arrange for care for Maggie's son, if required, for Maggie to get to these. She supports Maggie in setting her personal goals and helps her to record these in her personal health guide, which sits on the *HealthSpace* site, where Maggie can access it using a password.

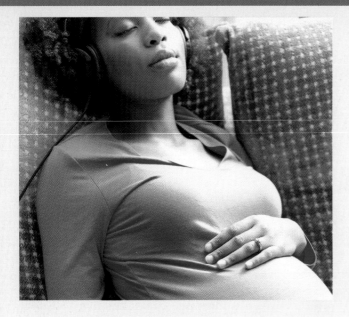

- determine what action they want to take and what support they can expect to get from the NHS and others to achieve this.

33. There will be natural points for people to review their health and develop their personal health guide:

- pregnancy;
- the birth of a child;
- entering and leaving school;
- starting work or entering further/higher education;
- a new year;
- a significant birthday as they get older;
- suspected or actual ill health;
- major life events, like bereavement, unemployment, entering a new relationship, or experiencing relationship breakdown; and
- preparing for retirement.

The NHS will provide help and support in developing guides, but can also help in putting them into practice – for example through specialised stop smoking services or the other health improvement and screening services outlined in Chapter 6.

34. Everyone will have help and support from the NHS, including from health trainers, if they want it but guides will be individual to each person and controlled by them. Our plans to develop health literacy and provide more and better health information in Chapter 2 will help people in developing the knowledge and skills to take that control and make their own guides. For children, the personal health guide will build on the child's health record and children's health guides discussed in Chapter 3.

35. If they want to, adults and children will also be able to develop their guide in an electronic form, linked to their *HealthSpace* on the internet. This will be an online personal health planning kit to develop their own personal health guide, based on who *they* are, what *they* want and what *their* circumstances are. This tool will help people to identify their own priorities for health and the changes that they feel ready to make, to receive online guidance about what will make the most impact on their lives and receive tailored advice on how to go about making changes and sticking to them. They will be able to include relevant material from their personal care records and create a selection of information and advice customised to their own needs. For example, a guide might include information about immunisations and contraception, as well as their progress plan on losing weight or stopping smoking.

Since its launch in 2003, a new user has opened up a *HealthSpace* account once every two hours – nearly 4,000 people. Patients have access to a new service called *HealthSpace*, a secure personal health organiser on the internet, at www.healthspace.nhs.uk. As facilities build up over time, people will be able to record more personal information and preferences in *HealthSpace* and make decisions on sharing information with the professionals who organise their care. The sort of information that it will be possible to record will be expanded and might include:

- access to NHS information services;
- graphing of variable personal data (weight, height, dietary intake, smoking, alcohol intake, blood sugar levels, peak flow readings; immunisation log and reminder service;
- location maps for NHS services;
- work with other NHS services: Healthy Living module (5 a day, give up smoking, etc);
- alert reminders; SMS appointment; and
- monitoring service (Self-Care and Expert Patient): diabetes and hypertension.

36. Online support will not be right for everyone and **the Department of Health will work to develop a number of tools for planning for health that will suit a variety of different needs and approaches.** Some people may prefer a health diary format, others a health personal organiser. What works for each individual will depend on their preferences and their goals.

CONCLUSION

37. Everyone would like to make manageable changes to improve their health, but people often want help and support to help them make and implement guides to do so. The new approaches set out in this chapter will help people by offering them the opportunity to develop their own personal health guides and providing access to NHS-accredited health trainers and other NHS and community resources to support them in acting on their plans for health.

38. The initiatives described in this chapter will ensure that there are opportunities for people to define and achieve their ambitions for health:

- Everyone will have access to an NHS-accredited health trainer. These trainers will help people draw up and review their health guides. They will also provide advice and support to help people choose health. They will also be able to help people identify and access other resources – from information to specialist services.
- Health trainers will be part of a wider workforce geared towards prevention of ill health and form part of a comprehensive health improvement service.
- The national competency framework for health will provide opportunities for people in the local community and voluntary sector to develop an understanding of health issues and allow them to develop health skills.
- People from all walks of life will get the opportunity to develop personal health guides, helping them take more control and enjoy better health.
- Each personal health guide will set out the contribution the NHS will make in partnership with the guide's owner.

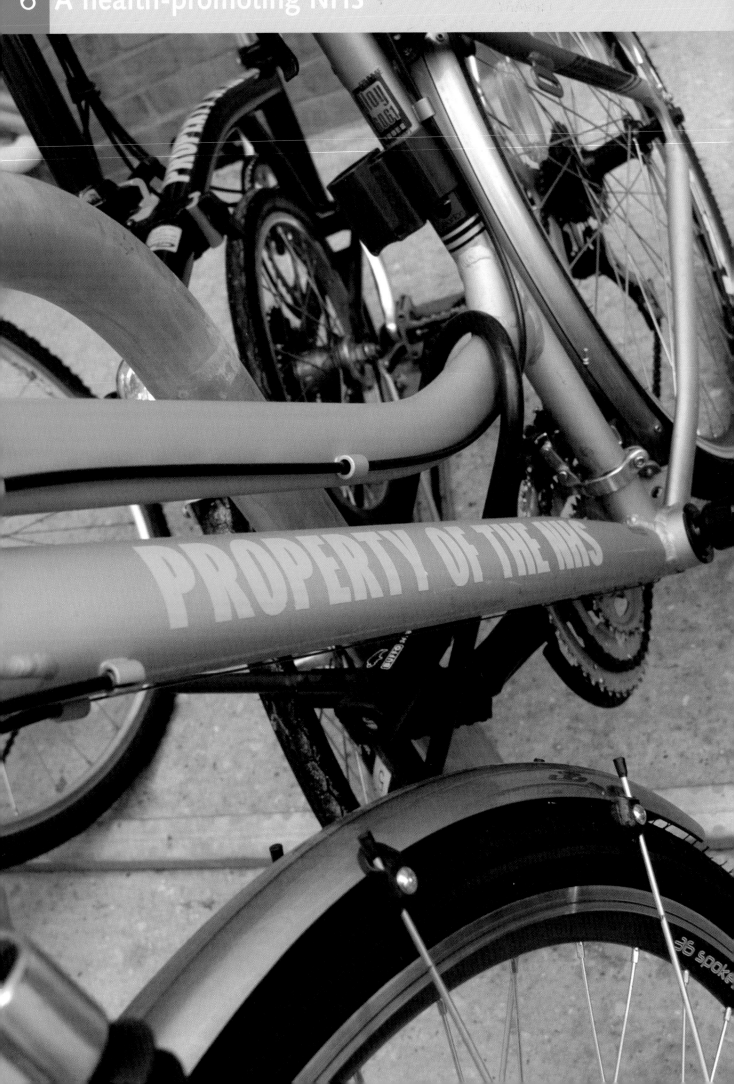

'Many of the benefits of engaging people in living healthier lives occur in the long term but there are also immediate and short-term benefits when demand for health services can be reduced, especially in those areas where capacity is seriously constrained.'

Derek Wanless

CHAPTER SUMMARY

This chapter sets out how the NHS, as it tackles waiting for treatment successfully, will increasingly become a health improvement and prevention service, supporting individuals in the healthy informed choices that they make. It includes measures to:

- *help local health services to plan and deliver effective action to tackle inequalities and improve health;*
- *make the most of the millions of encounters that the NHS has with people every week;*
- *ensure that all NHS staff have training and support to embed health improvement in their day-to-day work with patients;*
- *address the needs of people at particular risk; and*
- *ensure that health improvement and prevention services – such as sexual health services, NHS Stop Smoking Services, obesity services and alcohol services – benefit fully from the same drive for modernisation and improvement that exists across the rest of the NHS.*

INTRODUCTION

1. One of the founding principles for the NHS in 1948 was that it should improve health and prevent disease. After decades of underfunding, the Government's programme of historic investment and radical reform focused first on putting NHS treatment services on the road to becoming world class. Now is the time for the NHS to move on to become a true health service and not just a sickness service.

2. We need to invest in helping people to stay healthy. The public believe that the NHS should take a lead role in providing information, advice and support to enable everyone to lead healthier lives and prevent illness.[1]

3. This makes good economic sense too. One of the major choices facing society is how we can best use the £67 billion a year we now spend on the NHS, and make the most effective use of that new investment. Derek Wanless, in his two reports, drew out the financial consequences for a society that does not invest in health. If trends in obesity develop unchecked, or smoking rates stop falling, we will have to spend a growing proportion of NHS funds on coping with chronic conditions like diabetes and heart disease. The NHS will have to run ever faster to stand still. Derek Wanless made

1   www.kingsfund.org.uk/pdf/publicattitudesreport.pdf Opinion Leader Research survey.

CASE STUDY

'If England is to secure world-class standards of health, the enormous human, financial and physical resources available to the NHS need to be focused on the prevention of disease and not just its treatment.'

NHS Improvement Plan 2004

a powerful case for a new form of alliance between the NHS and society to halt these trends and become 'fully engaged' in promoting health. Action to support good health brings together the interests of individuals, the NHS and tax-paying society.

4. This chapter describes what the NHS will do to deliver on these aims. It describes the next steps to improve health, identify risk and prevent disease, by:

- ensuring that the one and a half million contacts people have with the NHS every day become opportunities for improving and promoting health;
- developing local services designed around the needs of local communities, with a particular focus on those in the most disadvantaged groups and areas; and
- developing the same systematic approaches to health *improvement* and *disease prevention* services that are already transforming NHS *treatment* services.

MEETING DEMAND FOR HEALTH BY PROVIDING CONVENIENT SERVICES

5. Chapter 2 set out how, in a new approach to health policy, the Government will lead a strategy for marketing health and some of the ways in which the Government will respond to raised demand for health. The NHS has a critical role in helping to match a new demand for health,

All patients with learning disabilities, registered at a large primary care centre in Warrington, were offered a health needs assessment and health action plans. A training programme was developed by two public health nurses to help staff deliver adapted mainstream services to people with learning disabilities. A year in to the project, 92% of the population had received an assessment compared with 22% the previous year.

"It was the first time in a long time that someone had asked me how I was feeling and what my worries for the future are. I feel like there is someone there now if I need advice."

Carer, aged 72

CASE STUDY

"Patients seem to prefer the informality of the walk-in centre which is less intimidating than the hospital environment," says lead nurse and centre manager at a new, out-of-hours, NHS Walk-In Centre, Southampton."

Green Light Pharmacy near Euston station in Central London not only provides 'typical' pharmacy services but has also transformed its basement into a local health education and meeting centre for local black and ethnic minority populations using Neighbourhood Renewal funding and private investment. It provides regular health education sessions to the Bangladeshi community, including specialist smoking cessation services.

The pharmacy also supports the *Skilled for Health* partnership for Bangladeshi people with diabetes by signposting into the classes and providing translation services. It also operates a training programme for community volunteers who encourage local people to complete a series of 'health risk assessment' questions which are analysed by the pharmacy and feedback provided on the patient's level of risk. The patient may then be asked to attend the pharmacy if they wish to have screening and a further opportunity to discuss healthier lifestyle options.

created by more information and effective national campaigns, with an accessible supply of practical opportunities and support for people to take action. In particular, people in deprived areas need to have good access to primary health care services. We need not just to tell people about what they can do to improve their health but make it convenient for them to follow through and sustain the changes that they want to make.

6. The NHS will play its part by building services around people's lives, and taking account of the different needs of different groups in the community, so that everyone can benefit. The aim is to put in place a reliable, effective and accessible infrastructure for health improvement and prevention services that matches the infrastructure for high quality treatment services that we all expect.

NATIONAL PLANS TO PUT HEALTH AND PREVENTION AT THE HEART OF EXISTING PROGRAMMES

7. The National Clinical Directors are already working with local clinical networks to drive through the improvements set out in National Service Frameworks (NSFs). These are delivering sustained improvements, building high quality services to treat and prevent conditions such as cancer, diabetes, coronary heart disease and mental ill health, and providing more integrated and effective care for children and older people.

CASE STUDY

8. In many cases, these already include a focus on prevention, such as several standards in the NSFs for coronary heart disease and diabetes, and the falls standard in the NSF for older people. And these have been backed by action. For example, the Healthy Communities Collaborative engaged older people in pilot areas working with professionals to minimise personal and environmental risk of falls in simple and practical ways. This led to a drop of 32% in the number of falls recorded by ambulance collection data over the one-year pilot.

9. But, as the Government and the NHS engage in a new approach to health policy, with new infrastructure and new action on health, existing health improvement and prevention approaches need to be adapted to maximise their impact and to mainstream a comprehensive approach to health improvement across the NHS from primary care, through hospital care to specialist services.

10. **Each National Clinical Director will work with clinical communities and networks to:**

- **identify where there may be scope to extend primary and secondary prevention in their clinical areas, including geographical variation in preventive action and prescribing rates;**
- **agree the most important steps to take, in particular to tackle health inequalities; and**
- **set how progress can be assessed.**

The Northern and Yorkshire office of Diabetes UK has successfully worked with local diabetes healthcare teams to organise and run 'Diabetes for Life' days in Leeds, Gateshead, South Tyneside and York. These events have each attracted around 150 people with diabetes, providing them with opportunities to better understand their condition, improve their health and get to know the range of local health and voluntary services.

The opportunity to talk to healthcare professionals in the informal setting and environment provided by the voluntary sector was invaluable for people who find it difficult to raise issues in ordinary clinical settings. These events have been led and organised by Diabetes UK but have relied on the full cooperation and participation of the local NHS.

Number of NHS contacts with the public every day	
Consult GP or practice nurse	890,000
Total community contacts	315,000
Out-patient attendances	122,000
A&E attendances	44,000
In bed as emergency admission to hospital	96,000
Courses of NHS dental treatment for adults	74,000
In bed as elective admission to hospital	38,000
NHS sight tests	26,000
NHS direct calls	18,000
Walk-in centres	4,000
Ward attendances	3,000

11. As part of this work, the National Clinical Directors with the Deputy Chief Medical Officer will make recommendations by March 2005 on how to build a comprehensive and integrated prevention framework across all the areas covered by the National Service Frameworks. Locally, primary care trusts (PCTs) will need to consider how far current arrangements for delivery of the NSFs meet the new framework.

MEETING DEMAND FOR HEALTH: LOCAL PLANS FOR CONVENIENT SERVICES

12. In order to make a difference, and to enable local health services to provide a strong infrastructure for health locally to meet increased demand for health, **we are giving PCTs the means to tackle health inequalities and improve health through:**

- **funding to give greater priority to areas of high health need. We shall continue and if possible accelerate distribution towards need and promote commissioning for health;**
- **new investment in primary care facilities for some 50% of the population by 2008 with a focus on the most deprived areas of our communities; and**

- **development of a tool to assess local health and wellbeing that will help PCTs and local authorities jointly plan services and check on progress in reducing inequalities: a health and wellbeing equity audit.**

Taking opportunities for health: the role of NHS staff

Evidence shows that:
- giving up smoking before an operation leads to faster wound healing and a shorter hospital stay;
- intensive individual support to give up smoking following a heart attack or heart surgery increases the likelihood of success;
- screening people who attend A&E in cases where alcohol is a potential cause, and offering brief advice on alcohol misuse, can help reduce re-attendance rates;
- referring older people who have fallen to a falls clinic can help prevent more serious injury at a later date; and
- a healthy diet and stopping smoking can contribute to healthy eyes and provides some protection against age-related macular degeneration.

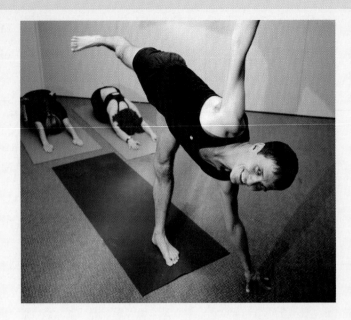

13. It will be NHS staff who put these plans into action and, to make a real, sustained impact, the whole of the NHS must join in. Across the NHS, there are one million interactions every 36 hours with people who are looking for some kind of help with their health. This offers enormous potential to get the right messages across. Every member of NHS staff has the potential to increase their role in raising people's awareness of the benefits of healthy living – as part of the wider NHS responsibility to patients to improve health, not just provide healthcare for the sick.

14. We will exploit this potential wherever we spot it. **As part of improving access and availability of tailored help to smokers wanting to quit we will, from 2006, offer NHS Stop Smoking Services on the new 'choose and book system'.** Choose and book is an electronic appointments service, initially for use by GPs in booking first outpatient appointments. From 2006, smokers will be free to choose available appointment slots for local NHS Stop Smoking Services, and book them through their GP practice. **We are also working towards embedding an offer of stop smoking advice as part of clinical assessment in surgical care pathways from 2006.**

15. NHS staff are among the most respected and valued people in England. People trust them and listen to them. This strategy will begin to provide

NHS staff with the support they need to make the most of that opportunity. This strategy marks the start of an important and fundamental cultural change in the way that the NHS relates to patients, with staff providing professional counsel and encouragement to patients on health, as well as high-quality treatment.

16. To support this change, **we will develop a National Health Competency Framework, which will include new programmes to give NHS staff the training and support they need to develop their understanding and skills in promoting health.** Through induction training for all new staff, undergraduate courses and continuing professional development we will equip all frontline staff to recognise the opportunities for health promotion and improvement, and use skills in health psychology to help people change their lifestyles. Elements of this training may also be helpful for workers outside the NHS, including in the voluntary and community sectors.[2]

Transforming health and prevention services

17. Health improvement and preventive services are patchy in quality and variable in coverage across the country. There is a geographical lottery in the support available. For a new approach to health policy in the 21st century, these services need to benefit from the same systematic drive

2   Annex B describes what we are doing to improve the evidence base, develop and disseminate information and best practice and improve training opportunities, learning from international best practice.

Tackling health inequalities: primary care is closing the gap, but more still needs to be achieved England

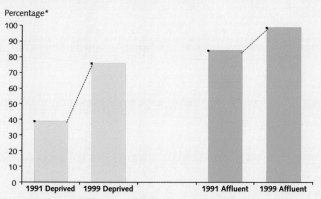

Percentage*

*Mean values of the percentage of GPs who achieved 80% targets in cervical screening, in two deprivation groups.

Source: D Baker, E Middleton, J Epidemiol Community Health 2003, 57:417-423.

CASE STUDY

for improvement and modernisation that is already transforming access to primary care, surgery and emergency care in the NHS. To meet increasing demand for health in the NHS, England needs fast, effective and universal access to high quality, people-centred health improvement and prevention services which have capacity to deliver.

18. We also need to tackle health inequalities head on, ensuring that the NHS provides people in disadvantaged areas and groups with services designed around their needs so that they want to use them. Developing new, innovative models of care and pursuing opportunities for sustained action as well as quick wins will be particularly important in tackling inequalities. We will need to ensure that service improvements do not increase health inequalities.

19. We will act on the best available evidence or develop new models of care to be evaluated in real time to determine what works ahead of wider roll-out. Health trainers will provide a key part of that infrastructure. Cultural change in the way that the NHS relates to patients, equipping itself to advise on health as well as treatment, will provide another. The rest of this chapter sets out how health and prevention services will be modernised over time, using the new health trainers as the foundation for an NHS where it is increasingly easy to get information and advice or access to services.

The Sheffield CIRC (citywide initiative for reducing cardiovascular disease) Programme aims to reduce inequalities in cardiovascular premature mortality. It delivers high-quality, secondary prevention programmes to an estimated 14,000 individuals with cardiovascular disease in the areas of highest need.

Fifty-one Sheffield GP practices received a tailored programme of support that included: training of nurses and doctors; additional nursing time; IT support; dietetics; physical activity and psychological specialist input. A citywide programme of user support and community engagement with ethnic minority communities also linked into the practice-based activities. Additional funding of £1 million has enabled the programme to be incorporated into the mainstream services of the four Sheffield Primary Care Trusts. By 2003, Sheffield had seen a 23% decline in the under-75 cardiovascular mortality rate in the most deprived fifth of its population since 2000, compared to a 16% decline in the Sheffield population as a whole.

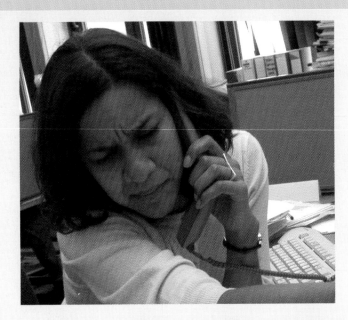

It describes what NHS organisations will do, and how they can work in partnership with local government and the independent sector.

20. In improving these services, we will initially concentrate on:

a. building a new local infrastructure for improving health, within the new arrangements for primary care services;

b. addressing the needs of people who face specific challenges:
   - making particular efforts to improve the health of people who have lifelong illnesses, particularly older people;
   - providing better support for people with mental health problems; and
   - promoting the health of people in prison.

c. tackling the big lifestyle issues:
   - maximising the effectiveness of NHS Stop Smoking Services;
   - improving services to help people who are overweight or obese and prevent overweight gain from an early age;
   - strengthening services to improve sexual health; and
   - delivering better services to prevent and treat alcohol problems.

AN NHS EQUIPPED TO MEET DEMAND FOR HEALTH

21. We will foster and expand a comprehensive range of community health improvement services that includes specialist practitioners who know how to:

- **help people develop their understanding and skills to improve their own health;**
- **strengthen community action for health to tackle inequalities; and**
- **work with communities, offering training, advice and support to a broad range of health professionals.**

22. As part of these changes, **new contracting arrangements for primary medical care, pharmacy[3] and dentistry[4]** are being introduced, to give more scope for PCTs to work with the health professions to shape services and introduce new providers to meet local need and local demand for health with high quality, professional services to support people in finding a healthy way of life.

23. For general practice, the new primary medical care contracting arrangements offer enormous potential to develop new ways to meet a growing demand for health, with more flexible services; greater choice; increased specialist activity; an improved range and quality of services; and services tailored to local needs.

---

3   From early 2005, subject to the conclusion of negotiations.
4   From October 2005.

CASE STUDY

In South London, the Rushey Green Health Centre has run a 'Time Bank' for three years. Doctors write prescriptions for medication but also for a regular hourly visit from a local Time Bank participant. This may be anything from help with the shopping to a friendly voice over the telephone. The Time Bank participants are also patients of the surgery and are happy to offer the care and support needed and earn their own Time Credits with the Bank at the same time. The doctors report that Time Bank participants visit them less.

24. In addition we will put in place measures which make the most of the contribution that pharmacists can make. Working at the heart of the communities that they serve, they have real opportunities to offer health messages and advice on issues such as diet, physical activity, alcohol, stopping smoking and looking after our own ailments ourselves. **The strategy for pharmaceutical public health, to be published in 2005, will demonstrate how pharmacists and their staff can contribute to improving health and reduce inequalities and how we can develop new services in the places they work.**

25. Many of the issues that affect people's general health are important for oral health too. **Under the new contractual arrangements for NHS dentistry, from October 2005 dentists will give a new focus to advice on the prevention of disease, lifestyle advice and the discussion of options for care.** They could, for example, work in conjunction with the wider primary care public health team to provide advice on smoking, and diet and nutrition – including prescribing sugar-free medicines where appropriate.

Maximising the reach of screening programmes
26. Each year the NHS offers health screening to about ten million people. The offer is of a specific screening test and it is for each individual to decide for themselves whether or not to accept it.

Screening programmes[5] do not operate in isolation; they have to be integrated with measures to encourage and promote the primary prevention of disease, and with the treatment services for those people who develop disease.

27. There is evidence of inequalities in take up of screening. As discussed in Chapter 2, the first step in influencing health behaviours in any group is to understand why people make the choices that they do, and the second is to design and deliver any new initiatives in consultation with them. PCTs will need to use health equity audits[6] to build a better understanding of why some people or groups are less likely to use the range of available opportunities for screening, and then act to promote take up.

SUPPORTING PEOPLE IN MAINTAINING THEIR HEALTH

About 60% of adults report some form of long-term or chronic health problem, including diabetes, asthma, arthritis, heart disease, depression, psoriasis and other skin conditions that can be controlled but not cured. Long-term conditions affect older people more than younger people. People in lower socio-economic groups are more likely to be diagnosed with more than one condition.

---

5   The screening programmes for individual conditions are grouped into four main programmes: the Antenatal and Newborn Screening Programme; Health for All Children – screening for children after the newborn period is integrated with a wide range of different measures to protect and promote health such as cancer screening; cardiovascular screening and diabetic retinopathy.

6   See Annex B.

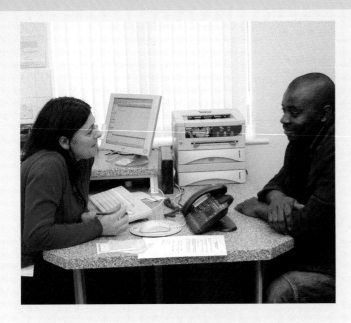

28. Health professionals need to consider the long-term benefits of encouraging patients to adopt healthy lifestyles even when advice on giving up smoking, exercising or changing diet is unwelcome and may initially make relationships difficult. For older, frailer people, who are more vulnerable to loss of independence and dignity, the right kind of support can markedly improve their ability to take ownership of planning and following through a healthy lifestyle.

29. The new arrangements in primary care will be important in helping people with long-term conditions or multiple conditions to make the most of their health. Most people with chronic diseases or disabilities are able to manage their condition themselves and to maintain reasonable general health with support from others. With help to develop their skills they can take greater control of their own health and their lives. The right support can often either slow the progression of the disease or reduce the problems of managing severe phases of illness.

The Expert Patient Programme supports people with long-term conditions to increase their confidence and improve their quality of life. Courses are designed to help patients develop skills in communication, managing emotions, managing daily activities, using the healthcare system, planning for the future and also improving their health through exercise, diet and ability to rest. Following the current pilot phase, we will make the course available through all PCTs by 2008.*

* The course will be available in a range of languages and media for people whose first language is not English and for people who may have sensory impairments or disabilities

30. **We will ensure that community matrons take the lead in providing personalised care and health advice with support from health trainers. By 2008, there will be 3,000 Community Matrons who will take on responsibility for case-managing patients with complex health problems.**

31. Giving health improvement advice can help people with chronic conditions improve their fitness and overall quality of life. Community Matrons will identify vulnerable people who are at risk or who would benefit from health advice to prevent deterioration in their condition, so that their needs can be better met, and the risk of deterioration or hospital admission can be minimised.

32. **Using proven best practice and modern information technology, local services will have the ability to provide targeted support. The Department of Health will advertise for independent sector partners to work with the NHS in a number of areas to develop new approaches to supporting health as part of self-care for chronic conditions linked to personal health guides.**

IMPROVING HEALTH FOR ADULTS WITH SOCIAL CARE NEEDS

33. The health needs of the adults who access social care will be the subject of further consultation in the preparatory work for the proposed Green Paper on adult social care. This has already identified action in line with the principles of this White Paper to improve adults' health and wellbeing.

PEOPLE IN PRISON

34. Generally speaking, people in prison have poorer health than the population at large and many of them have unhealthy lifestyles. Many will have had little or no regular contact with health services before coming into prison, and prison populations reveal strong evidence of health inequalities and social exclusion.

- The majority of prisoners are young and male.
- Most prisoners are in custody for periods of weeks or months, rather than years.
- Sixty to seventy per cent of them were using drugs before imprisonment and over 70% suffer from at least two mental disorders.
- It is estimated that at least 80% of prisoners smoke.
- Sixty-six per cent of all injecting drug misusers in the community have been in prison at some time, of whom half had been in prison before they started injecting.
- Male prisoners are much more sexually active in the community than the general population; all age groups having more lifetime sexual partners, and more partners in the year before entry to prison, than would be expected from the general population. They are also six times more likely to have been a young father.

35. Initiatives to improve health of prisoners offer a valuable opportunity to identify and tackle the wider health needs of a vulnerable and socially excluded population. They could, for example, be given information on health services and how to use them as well as information and support aimed at influencing their drug and alcohol and tobacco usage. Even if this did not persuade them to stop it might influence them towards less risky

CASE STUDY

"Many people with a severe mental illness experience considerable weight gain as a side effect of the anti-psychotic medication they take. They need dietary advice to deal with this. Some also live fairly chaotic lifestyles and need support to ensure that they eat regularly and healthily."

RETHINK 2003

behaviour, such as not injecting and adopting safer sexual practices.

> People in prison are being helped to stop smoking through services specially targeted to their needs, including access to Nicotine Replacement Therapy (NRT). These services are proving very successful. Early indications are that quit rates amongst prisoners, some 80% of whom smoke, are as good as or better than rates for other groups in the community. The initiative for prisoners grew out of a project between the Department of Health and the Prison Service. Learning from the project has been evaluated and disseminated to the field. Longer-term evaluation is taking place with prisons in the North West. Regional seminars have spread the learning widely across the NHS. This resulted in a set of 'transferable principles' being identified to reach disadvantaged smokers.
>
> *'Acquitted best practice guidance for developing smoking cessation services in prison'* Mark Braham, published Department of Health, 2003.

36. Some health promotion work has already been undertaken with prisoners. Results from prison smoking cessation programmes continue to be encouraging, with quit rates as good as, or better than, those in the outside community. The 'Walking the Way to Health' initiative, is being

Young people with psychosis who were previously 'missing' from mental health services in Plymouth are getting help from Insight, a local youth agency project which won a National Institute for Mental Health in England Positive Practice Award in 2003.

Sixteen to twenty-five year olds had been reluctant to access mental health services but now they wait at the doors at the Insight early intervention project, an integrated part of the Plymouth Youth Enquiry Service (YES). This aims to foster independence and inclusion in mainstream youth activities of those who are experiencing psychosis for the first time in their lives.

YES Deputy Director, Ruth Marriott, said, "Walking into a youth service used for social and leisure activity has a different feel to walking into adult mental health provision. Because the services on offer include sexual health, personal development and accommodation, as well as mental health, no one knows what aspect young people are accessing when they come in. This has helped to reduce the stigma attached to mental health issues.

"The focus is on all the issues that affect young people at this transitional time in their lives, such as housing, education and employment. We support them in making choices which have a positive impact on their mental health."

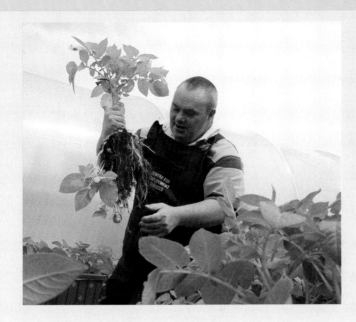

piloted in 10 prisons and promoting healthier eating and weight management proved a success in a project in a women's prison.

SUPPORT FOR MENTAL HEALTH AND WELLBEING

37. Transforming the NHS from a sickness to a health service is not just a matter of promoting physical health. Understanding how everyone in the NHS can promote mental wellbeing is equally important – and is as much of a cultural shift.

38. A coherent approach to promoting mental health needs to work at three levels:

■ **Strengthening individuals:** increasing emotional resilience through acting to promote self-esteem, and develop life skills such as communicating, negotiating, relationship and parenting skills.
■ **Strengthening communities:** increasing social support, inclusion and participation helps to protect mental wellbeing. Tackling the stigma and discrimination associated with mental health will be critical to promoting this increased participation.
■ **Reducing structural barriers** to good mental health: increasing access to opportunities like employment that protect mental wellbeing.

39. Other chapters discuss action to support families and children, and set out how strong communities and healthy workplaces can promote mental wellbeing. The NHS's distinctive contribution centres on the close contact that so many staff have with people at times when they may be vulnerable and in special need of support – new mothers, people coping with serious family illness or bereavement, people experiencing domestic violence, or people facing the loss of a job and the loss of self-esteem that can accompany that. We will ensure that standard one of the *NSF for Mental Health*, which deals with mental health promotion, is fully implemented.

40. The Department of Health will work through the National Institute for Mental Health in England (NIMHE) to ensure that day services for people with severe mental health problems develop to provide support for employment, occupation and mainstream social contact beyond the mental health system. This should include:

■ access to supported employment opportunities where appropriate;
■ person-centred provision that caters appropriately for the needs of all individuals, including those with the most severe mental health problems;

- developing strong links and referral arrangements with community services and local partners;
- providing befriending, advocacy or support to enable people to access local services (including childcare services);
- involving people with mental health problems in service design and operation; and
- a focus on social exclusion and employment outcomes.

Progress in service redesign will be monitored through the annual review of mental health services (the 'Autumn Assessment') by Local Implementation Teams. NIMHE will publish guidance for commissioners in early 2005.

41. As part of this work, we will ensure that the new training offered to NHS staff helps them recognise times when patients may be particularly vulnerable and strengthens skills and confidence to offer initial support and provide information on the sources of help that are available.

42. People with poor mental health tend to experience worse physical health than the rest of the population. Yet there is evidence that a healthier lifestyle will help improve not just physical health, but also mental health, mood and wellbeing. For example, regular physical activity reduces the risk of depression and has positive benefits for mental health including reduced

anxiety, enhanced mood and self-esteem. We need to do more to promote a more joined-up approach to NHS support for people with poor mental health. One early priority for NIMHE's anti stigma and discrimination programme is to address the physical health inequalities experienced by people with mental health problems.

> People with severe mental illness (SMI) are 1.5 times more likely to die prematurely than those without; partly due to suicide, but also to death from respiratory and other diseases. Depression is consistently been linked to mortality following a myocardial infarction; it increases the risk of heart disease fourfold, even when other risk factors like smoking are controlled for. People with severe mental illnesses also tend to have a poor diet; they are more likely to be obese; to smoke more; to access routine health checks less frequently, and get less health promotion input than the general population.

43. **We will use the lessons from a new approach being piloted[7] in eight centres in England to extend the new models of physical healthcare for people with mental health problems across all PCTs.[8]** Further development of this model will be linked into plans for providing NHS health trainers, outlined in Chapter 5, as health trainers may

7   New approaches to the management of physical ill-health among people with mental illness are being piloted by Lilly Pharmaceuticals.

8   Specialist teams, working in partnership with primary and social care providers, help support people with severe mental illness who are vulnerable to physical ill-health. The teams offer health checks and blood tests, guidance on diet, smoking and exercise, information for the patient and their GP, and the care worker, as well as ongoing support and follow-up. This approach can identify the early signs of disease, such as diabetes or coronary heart disease.

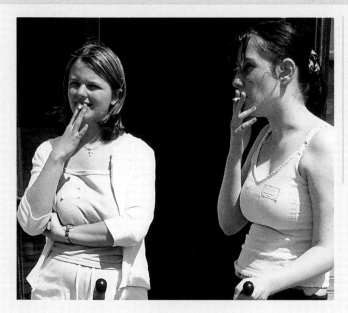

'Regular smokers who die of a smoking-related disease lose on average 16 years of life expectancy compared to non-smokers.'

choose to focus development of their skills in mental health or other specific areas.

44. We know that people who suffer from mental illness want more information about mental health and illness to help them manage their own care. **We will develop new approaches[9] to helping people with mental illness manage their own care and make available information for them on all aspects of health, both mental and physical wellbeing.**

45. For example, the report of the Social Exclusion Unit on Mental Health and Social Exclusion published in June 2004 sets out the action that central and local government will take, working together with different agencies, to strengthen support for people with mental health problems to access employment, as well as the education and leisure facilities that should be available for everyone. There are longstanding concerns about the quality of care and support provided to people from black and minority ethnic groups who have mental health problems. **The Department of Health is developing a programme of work to take forward the recommendations in *Delivering Race Equality: A Framework for Action*,[10] which outlined a whole system approach to tackle the inequalities experienced by people from black and minority ethnic communities in the mental health system of care.**

Support for smokers

46. Helping people to give up smoking remains one of the most important ways of preventing avoidable illness and death and reducing health inequalities. Studies have shown that smoking remains the most important cause of ill health in the most deprived areas. We have already set out our plans for action on information campaigns, for restrictions on smoking in enclosed workplaces and public places and for action on sales to underage young people. These actions will boost our wider, comprehensive tobacco control strategy, including the ban on tobacco advertising already implemented and new picture warnings on tobacco packets. The NHS has a special responsibility to back up all these measures with professional support to people who are trying to give up smoking, and to listen to what they want to help them quit.

47. Seventy per cent of smokers say they would like to be able to stop. Every year nearly three million smokers try to quit, although most find it very difficult because tobacco is so addictive. On average, ex-smokers have taken five attempts to quit for good. Achieving the national target to reduce smoking prevalence to 21% or lower by 2010 will not only depend on fewer people taking up smoking but also on large numbers of current smokers successfully quitting. If we hit our new

9   Evidence suggests that this can include electronic self-help options.
10 *Delivering Race Equality: A Framework for Action* consultation, published October 2003, available at: www.dh.gov.uk/assetRoot/04/06/72/29/04067229.pdf

Variation in NHS Stop Smoking Services across PCTs in 2003–04

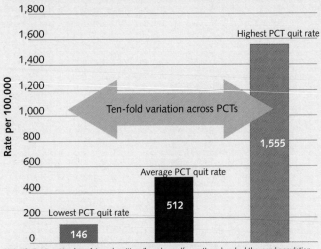

Note: Quit rate = Number of 4 week quitters (based on self report) per hundred thousand population aged 16 and over in 2003–04
Source: Department of Health and Office for National Statistics

Quitting method adopted	Number of smokers trying this method in each year	Success rate one year on	Number of smokers quitting through this route long-term
Willpower: no pharmaceutical or formal professional support	1 million	3–4%	30,000–40,000
NRT from shop or pharmacy	900,000	8%	72,000
NHS or other professional advice with NRT or bupropion (Zyban) through NHS (e.g. on prescription from GP)	600,000	8%	48,000
NHS Stop Smoking Services (with NRT or Zyban)	300,000	15%	54,000
Total	2.8 million		214,000

Source: Professor Robert West, Cancer Research UK

2010 target this would mean about 2 million fewer smokers in England as a whole, but with relatively higher numbers quitting in routine and manual groups where the target is to reduce prevalence from 31% in 2002 to 26% or less by 2010. We aim to increase the number of smokers who try to quit, and to support them to maximise their chances of sustaining success when they do.

48. Smokers choose a range of routes to try to quit. Most rely on willpower. Others also try without outside support but with the help of

Nicotine Replacement Therapy (NRT) purchased from a shop or pharmacy. Many get NHS help in the form of advice from a health professional, backed by NRT or bupropion (Zyban) (another stop smoking product) supplied under the NHS.

49. Willpower on its own is the least successful approach. There is good evidence that those who receive some formal support are more likely to succeed in quitting. We need to make it easier for people to access forms of help that we know are effective.

CASE STUDY

50. Increasing numbers of people are using NHS Stop Smoking Services, which provide more structured help for smokers who need or want it. These services use trained advisers to support smokers through the crucial first few weeks of a quit attempt (for example, with practical advice on how to cope with cravings) and help them to access and use NRT or Zyban to the best effect, along with the choice of one-to-one or group support. Since 1999, NHS Stop Smoking Services have helped over half a million smokers to give up for at least four weeks. However, there is currently an unacceptable tenfold variation between PCTs in the numbers of smokers successfully quitting per 100,000 population. These variations are in the numbers of smokers attracted to use the service, not in success rates once people enter a service. Some of the best services are in the most deprived areas. The most successful services:

- provide easy access through informal locations (community and leisure centres, pubs and clubs) at convenient times (eg outside working hours);
- encourage primary care contractors, and other NHS, community and workplace contacts to refer people to the service;
- identify and respond to special local needs, eg running mobile clinics in rural/isolated communities, providing services specifically for particular cultural groups; and

In early 2002, Hartlepool's first smoking cessation Drop-in Clinic was established at Greatham, a small village on the outskirts of the town. The success of this initiative led to the subsequent expansion of these community-based clinics across Hartlepool. Drop-in Clinics, staffed by Smoking Cessation Advisers working alongside Nurse Prescribers, offer clients an informal environment with easy access. They provide a holistic package of assessment, advice, information and a prescription of NRT with follow-up support and reviews.

Drop-in Clinics are run across Hartlepool. Perhaps one of the most unusual venues is the Fens Pub, where support is available on a weekly basis between 6pm and 8pm. The Fens Pub is within short walking distance of an area of the town which not only has a disproportionately high number of smokers (70% of adults in some pockets), but also some relatively profound levels of deprivation and health inequality (IMD national rank 25 in Owton ward). Up to 43 smokers wishing to stop have attended this clinic in a two-hour session.

The Drop-in Clinics create an atmosphere of understanding and non-judgmental support, which encourages those who fail to quit to ultimately return and try again. The target set by the DH for Hartlepool was to achieve 1,680 four-week quitters over a three-year period. The three-year target has almost been met within two years. Over 60% of those setting a quit date are smoke free at four weeks.

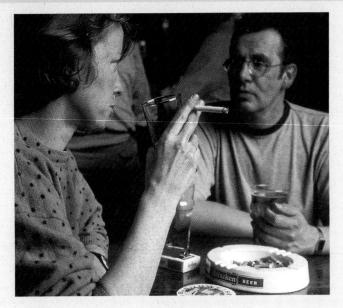

'We believe that an integrated and wide ranging programme of solutions must be adopted as a matter of urgency, and that the Government must show itself prepared to invest in the health of future generations by supporting measures which do not promise overnight results but which constitute a consistent, effective and defined strategy.'

Paragraph 153 of the Health Select Committee report

■ make good use of the media, linking to national campaigns like No Smoking Day, and adding targeted marketing for their local services.

51. We will now mainstream and resource this approach, and learn from what works best, driving improved performance through the system, and measuring for sustained success. We also need to gear up services to provide support to people who work in organisations which become smoke-free. New initiatives will need to be specifically targeted at routine and manual groups where the problems are greatest, and services tailored to reflect the needs of these groups. PCTs have a clear target to achieve in diminishing the prevalence of smoking and reducing inequalities and they will be performance managed against it; health trainers will provide extra capacity for stop smoking advice. To help them meet their target:

■ **In 2005–06, the Healthcare Commission will examine what PCTs are doing to reduce smoking prevalence among the local population, including their own staff, through tobacco control campaigns, championing smoke-free environments and provision of NHS Stop Smoking Services. Ongoing progress will be assessed against national standards and indicators.**

■ **We will establish a national taskforce to help increase the effectiveness and efficiency of the NHS Stop Smoking Services and provide practical guidance for local implementation,[11] in particular how to make services more people-centred.**
■ **We will identify and disseminate good practice on what works through Regional Tobacco Control Managers and the NHS.**
■ **We will develop pilots on using the electronic booking system to trigger advice for smokers on stopping, with a view to national roll-out.**

52. Although the formal NHS Stop Smoking Services may maximise smokers' chances of successfully quitting, not all smokers want to use them. We will expand the choice of help available and provide more support through alternative routes to meet smokers' needs.

53. We have piloted a new programme, *Together*, which offers ongoing help and support to smokers who want to quit. **We will develop the *Together* programme of support for smokers to quit and roll it out across England from Spring 2005 as part of the range of services that will be linked to Health Direct.**

11 This includes work with local authorities, all local NHS Trusts and community groups to identify opportunities for referrals to NHS Stop Smoking Services and the role of local clinical networks in prevention and championing Stop Smoking Services by increasing local referrals.

CASE STUDY

'Obese people, and the severely obese in particular, are more likely to suffer from a number of psychological problems, including binge-eating, low self-image and confidence, and a sense of isolation and humiliation arising from practical problems.'

Appendix Five, Paragraph 11, National Audit Office Report

The *Together* programme will offer smokers support through phone, e-mail and text in quit attempts. The pilot showed an increase in quit rates for those in the programme and very substantial increases among some groups.

---

54. We want also to widen the use and availability of NRT, which the National Institute for Clinical Excellence (NICE) as identified as among the most cost-effective of health interventions. However, NRT is not as readily available as we would like and both health professionals and smokers need to be more aware of how effective it is.

55. **We have a well-established partnership with the manufacturers of NRT, who have an important role in public health and in the promotion of therapies. In 2003 we agreed an innovative deal with the companies involved, under which they provide free NRT patches to PCTs in recognition of the increased investment the NHS is making in stop smoking products. This arrangement will increase the resources available to the NHS to help even more smokers quit.**

The Dorset 'Shape Your Life' programme was devised in 2002. Clients with a body mass index of over 30 with coronary heart disease risk factors and/or diabetes were identified from GPs' registers. If clients were sufficiently motivated, they joined a six-month weight reduction programme, with the aim of losing at least five kilograms. A wide range of options was offered, which included practice-based weight management groups, walking groups, commercial slimming organisations and Weight To Go at local leisure centres. Clients visited their practice nurse on a monthly basis to record weight and blood pressure and complete an evaluation form.

One hundred and forty clients have completed the programme across Dorset: 79% have lost weight, of whom 30% have lost five kilograms or more. Body mass index and blood pressure also reduced in the majority of clients.

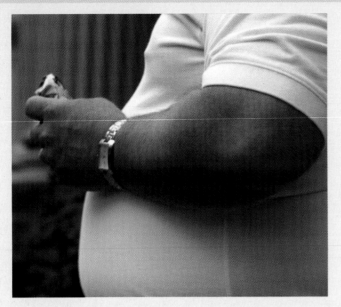

'It is difficult to separate cause from effect in the relationship between obesity and psychological disorders. Whilst mental wellbeing may suffer as a result of the pressures associated with being obese, psychological problems may equally contribute to the type of behaviours, such as emotional and binge-eating, that can result in the onset of obesity.'

Appendix Five, Paragraph 13, National Audit Office Report

56. **The companies have publicly committed to look at new and innovative ways of making NRT more widely available. They are currently discussing with the Medicines and Healthcare products Regulatory Agency (MHRA) the licensing restrictions around NRT, and are looking at wider access issues and other ways to promote the use of NRT, including:**

- **raising awareness among healthcare and related professions by committing resource to that work;**
- **new media campaigns;**
- **developing new and innovative therapies;**
- **promotion of therapies through a wider choice of outlets; and**
- **encouraging retailers to allocate more space for stop smoking therapy products and space alongside cigarettes.**

57. As part of the strategy outlined in Chapter 2, **we will extend our awareness-raising campaigns to promote the use of NRT for people quitting on their own or as part of an NHS-supported attempt.**

Better services to tackle obesity

In 2002, almost six out of ten women and seven out of ten men were overweight or obese. Balancing our calorie intake with calories we spend through physical activity is critical. Even eating an extra 10kcals a day can lead to gaining an extra pound in weight per year and gradually over the years this can become a significant problem.

'Overall, it appears that, over the past 20 to 30 years, there has been a decrease in physical activity as part of daily routines in England but a small increase in the proportion of people taking physical activity for leisure. Total miles travelled per year on foot fell by 26% and miles travelled by bicycle also fell by 26% (1975/6–99/01 National Travel Survey). This produced a difference of 66 miles walked per year between 1975–6 and 1999–2001. Twenty-five years ago we walked nearly three marathons a year more than we do now. For a person weighing 65kg this represents an annual reduction in energy expenditure equivalent to almost 1kg of fat.'

At least five a week: Evidence on the impact of physical activity and its relationship to health. A report of the Chief Medical Officer. Department of Health.

Understanding the lifestyles of different groups: prevalence of obesity in men and women aged over 16 by ethnicity (England 1999)

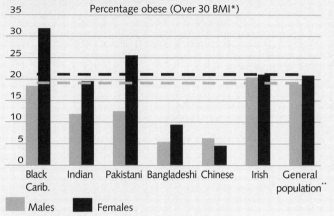

Percentage obese (Over 30 BMI*)

Males   Females

* BMI = body mass index
**It should be noted that the 'general population' refers to the entire population of England, and therefore includes minority ethnic groups.
Source: Health Survey for England 1999.

'The obesogenic environment needs to be tackled at the highest levels. It is not adequate to focus on the individual, especially the child, and expect them to exercise self-control against a stream of socially endorsed stimuli designed to encourage the consumption of excess food calories.'

Paragraph 176, Health Select Committee Report

58. Trends in diet and lifestyle over the last three decades have combined to bring an epidemic in obesity. More sedentary lifestyles, ready access to 'energy dense' food, an increased use of convenience foods, snacking and eating out, have all played their part.

59. In addition to the health risks – diabetes, heart disease and cancer – obesity can have far-reaching psychological and social implications for both adults and children, including reduced self-esteem, increased risk of depression, social isolation and lack of employment.

60. Action on obesity is not just a matter for the NHS: other chapters discuss the role of the food industry, food promotion to children, creating more opportunities for people to be physically active, and opportunities within schools. But a comprehensive response to the threats that obesity poses to individuals and society must include concerted NHS action. The aim must be as systematic and determined an approach to the prevention and treatment of obesity as to other signs/symptoms that signal high risk of disease, for example, high blood pressure.

Dr Foster survey of obesity services in the UK
The Dr Foster report concludes that:
- There is significant variation between areas in the UK in terms of primary clinical response to obesity and service provision.
- Action is focused on obesity as a risk factor for other chronic diseases rather than an illness in its own right.
- National initiatives to promote healthier behaviours – such as 5 A DAY and exercise on prescription – have been widely adopted and are now almost universal.
- There is more consistency around second line treatments (surgery and drugs) than first line.
- There is variation between areas in terms of services available and the communication of services to the public, the way in which the services are organised, and primary responsibility.
- There is scope for improved information for the public about schemes to tackle obesity – around 10% of areas said they did not provide any form of written information about services available.

Dr Foster website (www.drfoster.com)

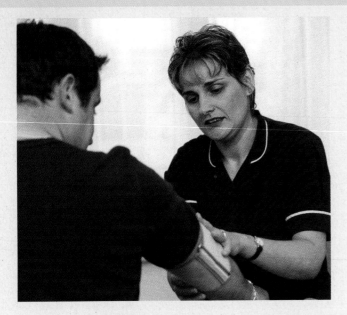

61. Recent studies[12] have found clinical services for obesity wanting, with significant variation across England. Although there are examples of good practice, preventive action is often taken only when obesity coexists with other chronic diseases, rather than as a clinical problem in its own right. Research[13] has found that there is a reticence among health professionals about raising the issue of obesity with patients, a lack of necessary skills to deal with obese patients, and a lack of clear referral mechanisms and services. Around 10% of areas did not have any written information about services available. There is a need for much improved information for health professionals and the public on how to prevent weight gain.

62. Children are particularly at risk and need a healthy start in life, but about 17% are now obese. We have introduced a national target to halt the year-on-year increase in obesity in under-11 year olds in the context of a broader strategy to tackle obesity in the population as a whole by 2010. The NSF on Children, Young People and Maternity Services includes action on obesity.[14] Chapter 3 outlines what schools and others will do to encourage healthy lifestyles in children and enable early identification and personalised help for those at risk of becoming overweight or obese.

Body mass index

Formula:

$$BMI = \frac{weight\ (kg)}{height\ (m) \times height\ (m)}$$

Classifications:

Body mass index (kg/m²)	Classification
Less than 20	Underweight
20 to 25	Desirable or healthy range
25 to 30	Overweight
30 to 35	Obese (Class I)
35 to 40	Obese (Class II)
Over 40	Morbidly or severely obese (Class III)

Source: BMI classifications from the Health Survey for England.

---

63. The basic messages about how to maintain a healthy weight by balancing energy in and energy out through diet and activity are clear. But there is currently less evidence about effective ways to help people who are obese or overweight to lose weight. Although we need better evidence, the urgency of the problem means developing, rapidly evaluating and implementing new approaches to managing obesity alongside research on what works.

64. We shall build on the good foundations already in place to implement the NSFs for coronary heart disease and diabetes. Guidance for PCTs on priorities and planning includes the need to give advice on diet and activity. The next challenge will be to act

---

12 Recent studies include those by the Health Select Committee and Dr Foster.

13 Report to the Department of Health – attitudes towards and practice of prevention in primary care: a qualitative study, OLR June 2004.

14 *National Service Framework for Children, Young People and Maternity Services: Key Issues for Primary Care* (September 2004) pages 11 and 12 www.dh.gov.uk/PublicationsAndStatistics/Publications/

CASE STUDY

on obesity as an issue in its own right using levers such as the new primary medical care contracting arrangements, including enhanced services and through negotiated changes which may be possible in the Quality and Outcomes Framework.

65. We have put action in hand to strengthen the evidence base on effective interventions. NICE has already carried out appraisals and published guidance on the use of drugs and surgery to treat obesity. **The DH has also commissioned NICE to prepare definitive guidance on prevention, identification, management and treatment of obesity and this is due to be available in 2007.**

CADISAP is a pilot scheme which is seeking to establish if culturally sensitive cardiac treatment and rehabilitation, designed around the needs of South Asian patients and their families living in the Waltham Forest area, can improve this population's health and quality of life. For the first time, it brings together teams from primary and secondary care to comprehensively manage treatment, support and education along the care pathway in a way which seeks to overcome some of the barriers which may prevent the South Asian population from benefiting from cardiac prevention and rehabilitation services.

Education about cardiac risk factors is provided along with psychological support, nutrition and weight management advice, support on taking lipid-lowering medication, increasing physical activity and blood pressure control. A gradual increase in periods of physical activity to at least 30 minutes most days of the week is encouraged, with practical support given, such as walking up the stairs rather than taking a lift, and walking to the shops rather than driving or taking a bus. Translation services are also available for those who need them.

The scheme, which is supported by the British Heart Foundation and the Department of Health, and partly funded by the Neighbourhood Renewal Fund, has already resulted in a high quit rate among current smokers, improved exercise capacity and changed dietary practices. A formalised, randomised controlled trial is now under way in the second phase of the scheme.

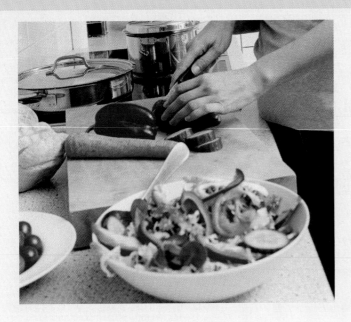

66. **We will develop a comprehensive 'care pathway' for obesity, providing a model for prevention and treatment.** A typical care pathway for a patient would involve:

> **Raise awareness and provide information**
>
> ↓
>
> **Raise the issue opportunistically and provide advice**
>
> ↓
>
> **Referral as appropriate to specialist service – to consider type of support required eg diet/physical activity; drugs; surgery**
>
> ↓
>
> **Review and maintenance of progress**

67. More specifically the prevention and treatment of obesity will ensure that:

- we have coordinated activity on obesity prevention and management in each PCT for both adults and children with a range of appropriately trained staff – to include health trainers, school nurses, health visitors, community nurses, practice nurses, dieticians and exercise specialists. Services may also be drawn from the voluntary and independent sector;

- there are clear referral mechanisms to specialist obesity services which will be staffed by multidisciplinary teams with specialist knowledge and training in obesity management (see paragraph 66); and

- in addition to specialist services there will also be trained staff who can work in different settings such as schools, leisure services and the community, working alongside obesity prevention and management experts within the overall whole system approach to obesity within a PCT.

68. **We will also commission production of a 'weight loss' guide, to set out what is known about regimes for losing weight and help people select the approaches that are healthy and are most likely to help them to lose weight and then maintain a more healthy weight.**

69. **We will commission further studies to support development of new approaches where there are gaps in the evidence base within the new framework for research discussed in Annex B. This will include production of specific guidelines for children's exercise referral.**[15]

70. **We will support the setting up of a 'national partnership for obesity'. The partnership will act to promote practical action on the prevention and management of obesity and as a source of**

15 In line with National Quality Assurance Framework for Exercise Referral Systems 2001.

information on obesity (for both diet and physical activity) and evidence of effectiveness.

71. The NHS will need to act on existing guidance and prepare to be ready to implement NICE guidance. The additional funding that will go to PCTs from 2006 will help them strengthen primary care capacity to prevent weight gain and tackle obesity, and to develop services to respond to patient needs across the whole care pathway.

Treatment programmes, including:
- regular weight checks for patients and advice on diet, nutrition and physical activity and weight loss by health trainers and other healthcare professionals;
- early identification of those at risk, eg opportunistic measuring of patients' BMI, followed by advice;
- local partnerships between the NHS, local authorities, schools and workplaces to deliver joined up action on nutrition and exercise;
- local initiatives on healthy eating– eg '5 A DAY' community pilots; and
- local interventions to promote activity across the population run by PCT, local authority and voluntary sector.

Treatment programmes, including:
- specific dietary and activity advice and exercise referral;
- behaviour change therapy geared to the needs of individuals, for example family-based action for children;
- long-term support for and review of chronic cases;
- targeted use of drugs and surgery where appropriate; and
- regular monitoring of progress and of related disease.

---

72. The number of people who are overweight and obese means that each PCT area will need a specialist obesity service with access to a dietician and relevant advice on behavioural change. PCTs do not need to commission all these elements from NHS providers, but should develop innovative clinical models that will help support evaluation of different approaches to delivery of obesity services at local level eg quality assured, commercial diet providers and leisure centres. Local partnerships with the voluntary and community sectors, local authorities, the leisure industry and other alternative service providers will be able to enhance capacity and the new primary care contracting arrangements support this. **The independent sector may have a key role in providing effective**

CASE STUDY

www.healthm8.net has been created by the Northamptonshire Healthy Schools Development Team, which works on behalf of Daventry and South Northants PCT, Northamptonshire Heartlands PCT, Northampton PCT and Northamptonshire County Council Schools Service. The website was designed in response to research which established that young people want an information source that is up to date, speaks their language, and is relevant and interactive. Young people and local partners have been involved in its development.

The site can be accessed anywhere that young people have the opportunity to use the internet, whether at school, at home, or in a cyber cafe, and they remain anonymous. It deals with subjects topic by topic. The sex and relationships section deals with building a relationship without feeling pressured to have sex; contraception; STIs; HIV and AIDS; confidentiality and where to go for help. The drugs section provides information about all categories of drugs, including prescribed and legal drugs and the law. It also deals with the consequences of taking drugs including their impact on health, travel, future opportunities and sport. Alcohol and smoking sections are also live. Healthm8 has an online agony aunt to answer any sensitive questions that young people may have.

Young people say that, "It's just what we wanted, it actually talks about sex!" and "It made us laugh, but got us talking". Teachers talk about the fact that, "It takes the pressure off of them having to introduce an embarrassing subject." Health professionals have welcomed the introduction of online confidential support for young people.

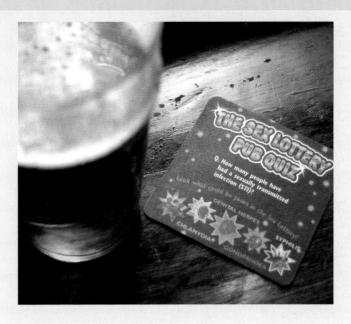

behaviour change programmes in ways that are more acceptable than traditional NHS care to some groups of patients. **We will test this as part of a procurement for a 'year of care' for diabetic patients.**

73. Another model we will test is to use the Healthy Communities Collaborative (HCC) principles in the prevention and management of obesity. This will build on existing HCC work on diet and nutrition, and accidents (see chapter 4).

74. **As part of the National Health Competency Framework we will allocate new funding for training, management, provision of evidence-based obesity prevention and treatment, based on National Occupational Standards for obesity.**[16] A priority will be to ensure that staff get the training they need.

75. We also need to help healthcare professionals develop more effective interventions.[17,18] **We will develop a patient activity questionnaire, which will be available by the end of 2005 to support NHS staff and others to understand their patients' levels of physical activity and assess the need for interventions, such as exercise referral.**

TRANSFORMING SEXUAL HEALTH SERVICES

HIV prevalence increased by 20% in 2002 compared with 2001

As many as one in ten sexually active young women under the age of 25 may be infected with chlamydia. If untreated, this can lead to pelvic inflammatory disease, ectopic pregnancy and infertility.

If a condom was used for every act of unprotected sex with a risk of an unplanned pregnancy or transfer of a sexually transmitted infection (STI), there would be a massive and immediate impact on the rise in STIs and HIV, significantly fewer unplanned teenage and other pregnancies and a reduced number of abortions.

76. Chapter 2 set out our plans for a major new campaign on sexual health. But information alone will not be enough. **We are committing new capital and revenue funding to tackle the high rate of STIs in England. This will support modernisation of the whole range of NHS sexual health services, to communicate better with people about the risk, offer more accessible services to provide faster and better prevention and treatment, and deliver these services in a different way.** This will need action to break down the boundaries between primary and specialist services, and new staff roles and skills. It is why

---

16 The Government is funding SkillsActive and Skills for Health – the sector skills councils for leisure and healthcare – to work together to produce common core modules of training on physical activity, diet and obesity which can form part of workforce training across all sectors. This work will be linked with the development of the new competency framework for health trainers discussed in chapter 5.

17 We are also consulting on making sport and exercise medicine a medical discipline.

18 Better and more timely information is needed to monitor trends and test the impact of action in all age groups. We will develop the Health Survey for England to monitor body mass index, and utilise data from primary care and schools, and the next round of National Diet and Nutrition Survey to achieve this.

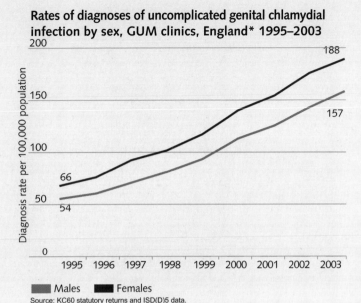

Rates of diagnoses of uncomplicated genital chlamydial infection by sex, GUM clinics, England* 1995–2003

Males   Females
Source: KC60 statutory returns and ISD(D)5 data.

National Standards, Local Action: Health and Social Care Standards and Planning Framework (2005–06/2007–08) includes improving sexual health within the national targets for the NHS and why sexual health will be included in the forthcoming round of Local Delivery Plans.

77. In future, sexual health services will be delivered through a flexible multidisciplinary workforce, in a range of settings, including:

- multidisciplinary teams headed by nurses linking between contraception, sexual health specialists (including genito-urinary medicine (GUM) consultants) and community, youth services and sexual health liaison workers working with primary care providers as part of a comprehensive range of services;
- extension of the roles of nurses, youth workers, community workers and pharmacists to include elements of sexual health;
- peer educators/youth workers trained to use the latest communications technology;
- mainstream primary care health programmes delivered by school nurses, health trainers, health visitors, community psychiatric nurses, midwives, and practice nurses;
- 'enhanced services' in the new primary medical care contracts; and

- more 'primary care practitioners with a special interest' working alongside sexual health experts in contraceptive, HIV and sexual health treatment services.

78. Services like testing and screening for STIs will increasingly be delivered in the community particularly targeting young people, vulnerable people and those who are hard to reach or at significant risk, such as black and minority ethnic groups. There are already excellent examples of good practice, but these are in small pockets and need to be expanded. The following models could form the building blocks for this expansion:

- one-stop shops combining treatment and prevention services;
- delivery of testing and screening in settings such as sports centres, supermarkets, shopping malls, workplaces, universities and community centres, at times and places which fit with people's lives;
- health buses, outreach workers, community pharmacies; or
- provision by the voluntary and commercial sectors.

79. We will have at the cornerstone of the drive for better sexual health a systematic campaign to reduce the incidence of **chlamydia**. Chlamydia can cause profound distress later in life through infertility or pelvic inflammatory disease.

High-volume testing for chlamydia is essential if we are to see an impact on rates of infection and the knock-on effect of ill health.

80. **We will accelerate implementation of a national screening programme for chlamydia, to cover the whole of England by March 2007**. The 1.2 million women who attend contraception services each year – the vast majority under 25 years old – will be the main focus for offering chlamydia screening as well as wider health advice. **We believe that the independent sector could contribute to providing efficient and convenient screening services. As part of the national programme we will take steps to introduce and evaluate the effectiveness of chlamydia screening in retail pharmacies starting in London.**

81. Prevention services also need to be developed and modernised. Contraception services have a key role to play in protecting against both unplanned pregnancies and STIs. To support this, the NHS will also strengthen the infrastructure for sexual health and contraception services in primary care. Currently contraceptive services are patchy and in some areas virtually non-existent. **We will therefore carry out an audit of contraceptive service provision in early 2005 and invest centrally to meet gaps in local services in particular to ensure that the full range of contraceptive services is available, good practice is spread and services modernised.**

82. Modernising the whole sexual health service will also involve transforming access to specialist treatment services. There is little point in screening people for STIs if they cannot also access specialist treatment quickly and easily. Current GUM services are struggling with the demands placed on them and primary care services need strengthening. **We are carrying out a national review of treatment services to provide advice and support on service modernisation for both commissioners and service providers and will follow this up with investment in both services and infrastructure.**

83. Delay in the detection and treatment of STIs promotes onward transmission, the development of expensive complications and the spread of HIV.

84. **We intend that the NHS should offer the same fast access to high quality GUM services that patients expect of other NHS treatment. The goal is that by 2008 everyone referred to a GUM clinic should be able to have an appointment within 48 hours** – a target that is currently only met for 38% of attendances.

CASE STUDY

A team at the Accident and Emergency Department of St Mary's Hospital, London have developed and validated the 'one-minute Paddington Alcohol Test' (PAT), a short screening questionnaire that detects those drinking excessive alcohol.

By auditing the use of PAT and selectively screening those who present with the 10 conditions most often associated with alcohol misuse, the department was able to increase the rate of detection of alcohol misuse four-fold.

People found to be consuming excessive alcohol are then offered an appointment with an alcohol health worker. Two-thirds of those offered an appointment accept the offer. If the appointment is on the same day that the person attends the A&E, 65% attend. In a randomised controlled trial examining the effects of referral, it was shown that those offered an appointment drank less alcohol during the following year than those who were not. People offered an appointment were also less likely to re-attend the department: for every two patients who accepted an offer of brief advice, there was one less re-attendance to the department during the following year.

Screening and referral for brief intervention for alcohol misuse in A&E provides an opportunity to help patients develop insight into the consequences of their drinking and promote improved health, thereby making best use of 'the teachable moment', i.e. the desire not to make themselves vulnerable again (reference – Crawford et al, The Lancet, 2004: 364: 1334–9).

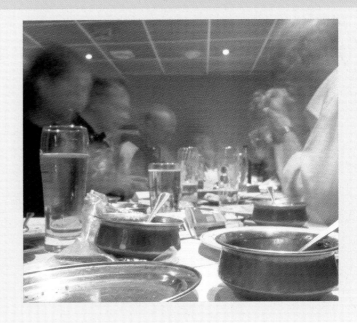

ALCOHOL

> Up to 35% of all accident and emergency attendances and ambulance costs are estimated to be alcohol-related. Alcohol misuse costs the NHS in England up to £1.7 billion each year.

85. While prevention interventions will provide the best means of tackling many alcohol-related problems, there is a small but significant number of people, particularly men aged over 30, who develop much more serious alcohol-related dependence or health problems. Left untreated these can lead to long-term ill health, including stroke and cancer, and premature death as well as placing a heavy burden on the families of those involved.

86. Alcohol treatment is currently provided by GPs and specialist addiction services but most of the 500 alcohol treatment services in England are located within the voluntary sector. These are usually funded by PCTs or local authorities and receive referrals from GPs or other NHS specialists.

87. The cross-government Alcohol Harm Reduction Strategy for England recognised that the provision of alcohol treatment in England was patchy and that some areas were unable to provide access to the full range of support needed.

By April 2005:

■ the DH will publish national and local audits of the demand for and provision of alcohol treatment.

By May 2005:

■ the National Treatment Agency (NTA) will publish 'Models of Care' guidance on the organisation of alcohol treatment and a road map detailing how to put this into practice.

88. These will lay the foundation for the future development of alcohol treatment within England. However, it is already clear that in order to provide high-quality, local services suited to the needs of service users, their families and carers, many areas will need long-term improvements in their current provision. To support this we will build on the commitments within the Alcohol Harm Reduction Strategy for England through:

■ **guidance and training to ensure all health professionals are able to identify alcohol problems early;**
■ **piloting approaches to targeted screening and brief intervention in both primary care and hospital settings, including A&E departments;**
■ **similar initiatives in criminal justice settings with the aim of reducing repeat offending, by ensuring that alcohol treatment needs are met alongside drug misuse treatment needs;**

- **developing a programme for improvement for alcohol treatment services, based on the findings of an audit of demand for and provision of alcohol treatment in England and the *Models of Care* Framework for alcohol treatment.**

These initiatives will be supported, from April 2006, through additional funding provided through the Pooled Treatment Budget for Substance Misuse.

CONCLUSION

89. The commitments in this chapter set out a starting point for ensuring that the NHS is as well placed to meet demand for health as it is for meeting demand for treatment. It puts in place the foundations for:

- national and local NHS service planning and commissioning arrangements which recognise the needs of all parts of the population and develop services to focus improvement in areas with the worst health outcomes;
- a comprehensive, accessible and high-quality set of health improvement services available in all communities;
- new models of contracting for primary care will mean easier access to health improvement advice especially for those who find it hardest to obtain this now;

- all NHS staff being able to give appropriate advice on basic health and lifestyle issues, promoting physical and mental wellbeing;
- linking health improvement advice to routine clinical practice;
- access to high-quality NHS Stop Smoking Services in all areas;
- the NHS offering real practical support on healthy eating, exercise, weight gain, clinical treatment for obesity, and a strong focus – with partner organisations – on prevention;
- accessible sexual health services delivered in both community and hospital settings;
- chlamydia screening available across England by March 2007;
- 48-hour access to a GUM clinic by 2008; and
- NHS health professionals able to identify problems with alcohol and provide brief interventions in A&E settings.

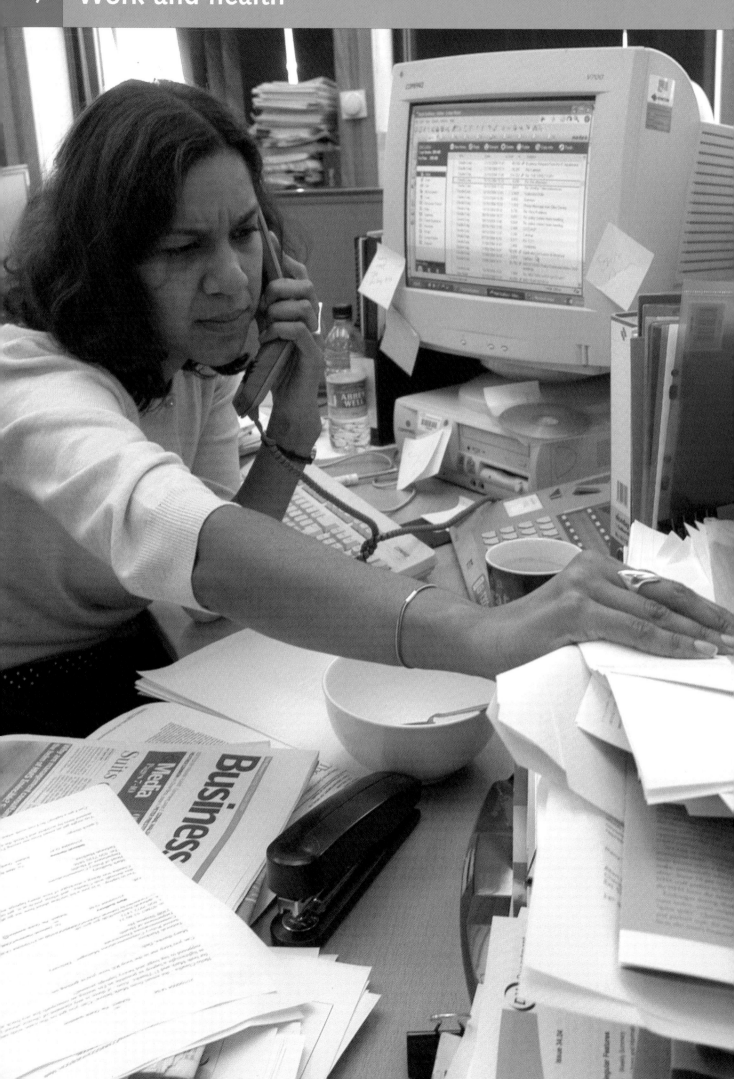

CHAPTER SUMMARY

For people in employment, work is a key part of life. The environment we work in influences our health choices and can be a force for improving health – both for individuals and the communities they are part of. Work offers self-esteem, companionship, structure and status as well as income.

This chapter sets out the action that employers, employees, Government and others can take to extend healthy choices by:
- *reducing barriers to work to improve health and reduce inequalities through employment;*
- *improving working conditions to reduce the causes of ill health related to work; and*
- *promoting the work environment as a source of better health.*

It also sets out what the NHS will do to become a model employer in supporting and promoting the health of its 1.3 million staff.

EMPLOYMENT FOR HEALTH

1. Work, and the rewards it brings, allows full participation in our society. It also leads to better health, particularly mental health. On the other hand, being out of work leads to poorer health and a shorter life.

2. Throughout this White Paper we have emphasised the importance of people making healthy choices, and the relationship between those choices and their environment. Work is a very important part of that environment. Having a job, and having a job in a healthy environment, will improve or hinder your chances of making healthy choices. These issues cannot be controlled by individuals, but need support from Government, business and trades unions. This chapter therefore combines individual action with the importance of interventions by powerful institutions to improve health.

3. The Government has already done much to increase the number of people in employment. Since 1997, the number of people in work is up by 1.9 million.[1] What has become clear through policies such as the New Deal is that personal services built around the needs of individuals are essential to encourage people back to work.

1   Office for National Statistics.

CASE STUDY

In 2004, London First established a Health Champions group, with members from a range of sectors including property developers, city law firms, higher education, health insurance and Strategic Health Authorities (SHAs). The group has devised a Wellness Index (aka The Company Doctor) which comprises a number of indicators that reflect the inextricable link between the 'health' of a business and the health of its employees. The aim is to use these indicators to track London business' health improvement over time.

4. Employment levels are at their highest rates ever. But significant numbers of people are out of work on the basis of a health condition or disability – around 7.5% of the working age population. Many of those who are currently not economically active might benefit from being in employment.

- The Social Exclusion Unit report *Jobs and Enterprise in Deprived Areas* contains new evidence about local pockets of unemployment and low economic activity that exist across the country and sets out what more the Government will do to make sure the benefits of full employment are felt in every neighbourhood in England.
- *Building on New Deal: Local Solutions Meeting Individual Needs*[2] sets out how we will continue to develop New Deal to help more people, particularly those who face specific barriers to entering, remaining in or progressing in employment because of disability, health conditions, childcare responsibilities, age, language or skills problems.

493,000 young people have moved from the New Deal into work and, without New Deal, long-term youth unemployment would have been twice as high. New Deal 50 plus, along with Working Tax Credit, has helped over 1,100,000 older people move into work with additional financial assistance. And 261,000 lone parents have moved into work through New Deal.

- The *Age Positive Campaign* promotes recruitment and retention of older workers as part of an age diverse workforce. The Government will outlaw age discrimination in employment and vocational training by December 2006 in line with the EU Directive on equal treatment.
- The Social Exclusion Unit report *Mental Health and Social Exclusion* identifies employment as a critical issue for action – 900,000 people with mental health problems form the largest group of disabled people currently on benefits.

Returning to work after sickness

5. A common view, sometimes inadvertently reinforced by health professionals, is that people with a physical or mental health problem should not try to go back to work until they are fully recovered. But with many conditions inactivity compounds poor

2   Department for Work and Pensions, June 2004.

health and leads to long-term absence from work.
There needs to be wider recognition of the positive
benefits for individuals and their employers that can
come from getting people back to work when they
have been off sick. For people who can be helped
back to work again, a job can itself be an important
step in the road to recovery and rehabilitation, helping
people to enjoy better health and well-being as well
as giving them greater control over their own health.
And being out of work for long periods of time is
likely to make a person's health problem much worse.

Unemployment is an important determinant of
inequalities in the health of adults of working
age in Britain, with people lower down the social
scale being hardest hit. Adverse effects
associated with unemployment include:
- increased smoking at the onset of
  unemployment – the prevalence of smoking
  is considerably higher among those who
  are unemployed;
- increased alcohol consumption with
  unemployment, especially in young men;
- more weight gain for those who are
  unemployed;
- reduced physical activity and exercise;
- use of illicit drugs in the young who are
  without work;
- increased sexual risk-taking among
  unemployed young men; and
- reduced psychological well-being, with a
  greater incidence of self-harm, depression
  and anxiety.

CASE STUDY

The number of people claiming incapacity benefit has trebled between 1979 and 1997 from 700,000 to 2.4 million. The Government pays out £13 billion a year on incapacity benefits. Most of those on incapacity benefits have conditions such as depression, musculoskeletal problems and cardio-respiratory problems (such as angina) – conditions which, in most cases, can be managed effectively with the right advice and support from the health community.

The longer someone is signed off, the less likely they are to return to work. For example, those off sick with back pain for six months have only a 50% chance of returning to work; after a year, that chance reduces to 25%.

CSAG report on back pain, 1994.

6. People are often apprehensive about returning to work. We are encouraging employers to use temporary job modifications to help people back – even if they are not able to do their usual job. This can be of benefit both to employees, in terms of longer-term health, and to employers, who will not lose an experienced worker and face the costs of replacing them.

Since 1995, South West London and St George's Mental Health NHS Trust has successfully increased its employment rate for people with severe and enduring mental health problems. The Trust has developed a Vocational Services Strategy based on the individual placement and support approach. Occupational therapists and borough mental health and employment coordinators work within clinical teams to enable people with severe mental health problems to access open employment and mainstream education. Ongoing support is included in care plans, with a focus on individual choice. After one year, the employment rate rose from 10% to 40%, and the percentage not engaged in education, training or employment dropped from 55% to 5%. In 2003/04, the Trust supported 271 people into open paid employment.

CASE STUDY

During National Men's Health Week 2004, Hassocks Health Centre ran an 'MOT' clinic next to the railway station between 5.30 and 8pm. Almost 70 men attended for blood pressure, cholesterol and diabetes tests as well as body mass index assessment. Many of the men commented that they did not visit the Health Centre because it was open only from 9am to 5pm and they did not want to 'bother' the staff by requesting a check-up if they did not actually feel unwell.

7. For people with mental health problems, the biggest obstacle to returning to work is often fear of stigma and discrimination by their employers. Fewer than four in ten employers say they would recruit someone with a mental health problem.[3] In June 2004, we launched a new anti-stigma strategy *From Here to Equality*. **The National Institute for Mental Health in England will work with the Disability Rights Commission to challenge discrimination against people with mental health difficulties, and enable more to gain access to employment.**

The Prime Minister's Strategy Unit has been asked to carry out a project to assess the extent to which disabled people are experiencing adverse economic and social outcomes in the UK; to identify why this is happening and what are the implications; and to assess what can be done to improve the situation. The project has highlighted the multi-faceted links between impairment, ill health and a range of socio-demographic factors, many of which are addressed in this White Paper. It has suggested that there should be a high-level debate among health professionals about ways in which work can feature more strongly as a positive driver for good health. A final report from the project will be published.

*The "Improving the Life Chances of Disabled People" project was announced in December 2003, and published an Interim Analytical Report in June 2004. Further information is available at www.strategy.gov.uk/output/Page5046.asp. Braille versions of publications are also available. Contact: Strategy Unit 'Disability' Team, Cabinet Office, Room 4.14 Admiralty Arch, The Mall, London, SW1A 2WH, Disability@cabinet-office.x.gsi.gov.uk

3   SEU report on mental health and social exclusion.

CASE STUDY

Yvonne, aged 57, had been a teacher all her working life. However, following instances of bullying at work she became clinically depressed (medicated) and felt she was not able to go back to the classroom. She retired on health grounds and felt at the age of 56 that she would never work again. Her family and friends rallied round and, although it helped to have their support, it did not alleviate the stress and depression she was feeling. Her personal adviser, Chris, discussed attending a pilot course, 'Help for Health', run at the local hospital. The group therapy sessions, run over six afternoons and based on a mixture of cognitive behavioural therapy, relaxation, etc, were, in Yvonne's words, "the very last resort". After assessment and attendance on the first session, she decided she would not be attending again as it was too uncomfortable to talk to strangers about her feelings. However, as the second week neared she decided to give it another go; when she arrived all the other group members told a similar story.

Yvonne and the others appreciated the support of other group members as much as the support of the psychotherapist running the sessions as they could relate to each other's problems and potential solutions. Six weeks later, having identified that she could take her hobby of floristry to another level, she enrolled on a self-employment course, again through her adviser. Yvonne launched her business, 'Aquilegia', on 29 September and couldn't be happier.

Pathways to Work pilots are helping much greater numbers of people on incapacity benefits get themselves back to work and improve their health. In these pilots, there is increased support from specially trained advisers in Jobcentre Plus, financial incentives and a Choices package. Where continuing health problems pose a significant barrier to getting back to work, the local NHS is working closely with Jobcentre Plus to help people manage their health and return to work. Early results suggest this approach is successful.

---

8. The Department of Health (DH) will work through the National Institute for Mental Health in England and in liaison with the Department for Work and Pensions (DWP) to implement evidence-based practice, in particular Individual Placement Support. This will include working towards access to an employment adviser for everyone with severe mental health problems. Provision of vocational and social support will be embedded in people's treatment plans and will include:

- establishing employment status on admission to hospital, and supporting job retention;
- promoting involvement of carers and families;
- identifying a lead contact on vocational and social issues in secondary healthcare teams;

- strengthening links to key local partners, in particular Jobcentre Plus and education providers; and
- access to advice and support on benefits issues.

9. Healthcare is about returning patients to good health, and that includes getting them back to work. Health professionals, wherever they work, need to start from the point of view that getting people back to work is likely to benefit their long-term health. Return to work must be seen as the norm and, where appropriate, should be included in treatment plans from the outset. Primary care trusts may want to consider developing a championship role for health professionals who are equipped to advise their colleagues on occupational health issues and share good practice in supporting return to work.

10. There are many barriers to retaining, regaining or accessing work. The Government is determined to show leadership in this area. We recently published a *Framework for Vocational Rehabilitation*, which is the first step towards developing a new approach to helping people back to work following injury, illness or impairment.

11. Expansion and diversification of the NHS will ensure access to services in a way that fit better with people's working lives. More people already have the option of accessing healthcare through NHS Walk-in Centres near their place of work or through NHS Direct, as well as through their GP.

IMPROVING WORKING CONDITIONS

Two million people suffer an illness they believe has been caused by, or made worse by, their work.

12. Although being in work generally leads to better health, not all workplaces are healthy. There is persuasive evidence that a lack of job control, monotonous and repetitive work, and an imbalance between effort and reward are associated with a higher risk of coronary heart disease and other health problems. And, although work is generally good for people's health, poor health and safety management increases the risk of occupational diseases and injury. 'Bad' jobs may make people ill.

The Whitehall II Study concluded that job strain, high job demands and, to some extent, low decision latitude are associated with an increased risk of coronary heart disease among British civil servants.

CASE STUDY

Leeds City Council set up a health and safety risk-assessment training forum to raise awareness of workplace risks in the small and medium-sized enterprise (SME) sector. Information was provided about the costs of accidents and occupational ill health to SMEs and the UK as a whole, and how to facilitate improvements in the well-being of employees by encouraging a more positive health and safety culture. In addition, sources of self-help and support services were provided. The forum consisted of seven training sessions, the material from which has been incorporated into a free CD-ROM that can be used as a stand-alone training package.

Health and safety at work

13. A key driver of the Health and Safety Commission's new strategy is making advice and support more accessible and getting workers more involved in taking decisions that affect their health and safety.

The Health and Safety Executive's (HSE's) *Constructing Better Health* (due to launch in October 2004) is an occupational health support pilot for the construction industry. The scheme is being led by the construction industry, with Government providing a contribution to funding. This pilot includes health risks education and awareness-raising, free on-site risk assessments for employers and occupational health screening for workers. The pilot will also provide a 'gateway' to further specialist support, if required.

14. Many small and medium-sized employers are concerned about contacting HSE or local authorities for advice and information. This means that those who could most benefit are not accessing a body of knowledge on industry best practice and expert information. HSE is putting in place a programme of actions to help companies implement best practice as they work towards implementing their *Strategy for Workplace Health and Safety in Great Britain to 2010 and Beyond*.

Stress at work

> Stress-related conditions and musculoskeletal disorders are now the commonest reported causes of work-related sickness absence.

15. A complex range of issues around work can act as a cause of mental illness. Often this is described generically as stress. Many people are concerned that stress at work affects people's well-being. But some level of stress is often a normal part of everyday life. It is excessive pressures in the workplace, often in combination with stress or pressures in our social life, that can reduce our sense of mental well-being and, in some cases, lead to physical and mental ill-health.

16. A focus on individual stress can be counterproductive, leading to a failure to tackle the underlying causes of problems in the workplace. Evidence has shown that poor working arrangements, such as lack of job control or discretion, consistently high work demands and low social support, can lead to increased risk of coronary heart disease, musculoskeletal disorders, mental illness and sickness absence. The real task is to improve the quality of jobs by reducing monotony, increasing job control and applying appropriate HR practices and policies – organisations need to ensure that they adopt approaches that support the overall health and well-being of their employees.

> 3.74 million workers clock up more than the 48-hour limit under the Working Time Directive – 423,000 more than in 1992 when there was no long hours protection (Labour Force Survey, Department of Trade and Industry.
>
> The Government introduced the Work–Life Balance campaign in 2000. The campaign aims to help employers recognise the benefits of adopting policies and procedures that enable employees to adopt flexible working patterns. This will help staff to become better motivated and more productive because they will be better able to balance their work and other aspects of their lives. Four years on, there is evidence that employers offering flexibility in working arrangements are experiencing an increase in recruitment and retention, employee commitment and productivity, and a decrease in staff turnover and sickness absence. A report by the Institute for Employment Studies shows some small businesses save up to £250,000 on their budget, simply by using family-friendly work policies. One company claimed profitability was up by 37%.

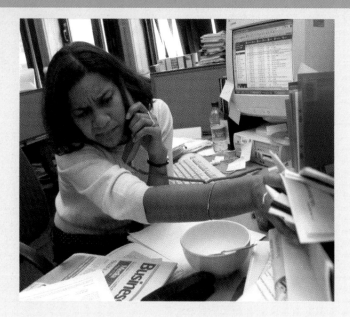

17. HSE has recently published (2 November 2004) new management standards for stress in the workplace.[4] These materials have been developed to help employers manage the risks of stress, following consultation with a wide range of stakeholders.

Occupational health support

Forty million working days are lost each year to occupational ill health and injury. Of this figure, 33 million are due to occupational ill health.

While many people working for large organisations do have access to occupational health support, very few of those working in small companies are provided with access to such support. Some research suggests that the percentage of small companies providing occupational health support could be as low as 6%, and as little as 2% for micro companies.

CRR 445/2002 Survey of use of occupational health support, *Health and Safety Statistics Highlights 2002/3*, HSE. 2003.

18. There are many providers of occupational health support in the public, private and voluntary sectors. In 2001 we launched NHS Plus, a network of about 100 occupational health departments in the NHS to increase occupational health support for other employers. Research shows that, although its work has grown at a rate of around 20% a year, more needs to be done. We will increase the availability of NHS Plus services in parallel with the development of occupational health services in the NHS. **We are working to develop evidence-based guidelines on occupational health and we will bring forward measures to ensure that services are of a consistently high quality. SHAs will be asked to demonstrate how development is progressing in their areas.**

On 27 October, HSE launched a 'best practice approach' to help employers and managers, in partnership with their employers, to manage proactively long-term sickness absence and help those off work sick, whatever the cause, to return to work. To support this, HSE has also produced a best practice guide for employers and managers, a free desk aid for SMEs, a free leaflet for employees and new HSE web pages.

CASE STUDY

19. Occupational health is a matter for all health professionals. Our aim is to build a three-way partnership between health professionals, individuals and employers. **To help ensure that employees are able to return to work as soon as possible following injury or illness, we will ensure that the NHS supports a wider occupational health approach. The medical Royal Colleges and faculties are working on ways to put this into practice in both primary and secondary care.**

Sickness absence costs employers at least £11 billion each year – this is 16% of salary costs.

■ Swiss Re* research has found that 90% of employers believe sickness costs can be significantly reduced, yet very few employers monitor sickness absence or take active steps to reduce it.

  – 55% of employers do not measure the cost of sickness absence.

  – Only 49% of employers have set targets to reduce sickness absence.

  – 50% of businesses do not offer occupational health services.

■ However, 60% of employees do want employers to take some responsibility for their healthcare.

* Swiss Re is a global reinsurance company.

The *Everyday Sport* campaign was launched in June 2004 to encourage people in the North East to become more active. The region was specially selected for this four-month test case because it has some of the lowest levels of participation in physical activity and sport in the country. Using TV and outdoor poster advertising, supported by a host of local media competitions and stories, the campaign encouraged citizens to do a little more activity each day in a way that suited them. Hundreds of organisations took part and staff tackled lazy lifestyles by getting involved in a range of activities such as speed walks at lunch time, Everyday Sport Office Games and team activities after work.

"Everyday Sport activities are ideal because they are easily accessible to large numbers of staff and show that being active doesn't have to be complicated. Something as simple as taking the stairs instead of a lift can contribute to a healthier lifestyle, and we are just as happy to say 'best foot forward' rather than 'mind the doors,'" commented David Hood, Assistant Director, Corporate Responsibility, from Northern Rock in Gosforth.

CASE STUDY

The Broadgate Centre in the City of London was redesigned with fitness in mind. It is one example of a new generation of 'fit' office buildings being designed by architects to encourage employees to become healthier by making them walk while they are at work. The design policy is for fitter people and a fitter environment. Meeting rooms, canteens and car parks are being put at appreciable distance from desks so workers have to expend energy getting to them.

PROMOTING HEALTH IN THE WORKPLACE

20. A large proportion of the population is employed and spends more than a third of its waking hours at work. If the workplace enables and supports health, employees are more likely to make healthier choices. For many people, the work environment constrains the choices available and makes it difficult to choose health. Central government departments can show the way here. **Sport England will provide a free consultancy service to government departments on how they can encourage and support staff to be more active in the workplace.**

The Health and Safety Executive (HSE) is developing innovative partnerships, in the public and private sector, to provide occupational health, safety and rehabilitation support (OHSRS).

The ultimate aim is for a support service that offers employees and employers advice on best-practice solutions for assessing and reducing exposure to key health risks, with a gateway to further specialist support if required. It would help employers to employ and retain those in poor health or disabled and ensure that work does not harm their health.

Pilots are already planned or under way that will test HSE's basic model for support, for example in the construction industry and in the Kirklees region. In addition to these pilots, funding has been allocated for further pilots to test the impact of the model for delivering occupational health and safety support. Evaluation of these pilots will provide essential information to identify best practice in changing behaviour and establish the financial model necessary to provide a sustainable scheme with national coverage.

21. Many employers recognise that they have a direct interest in creating an environment that helps people make healthy choices: because of

CASE STUDY

corporate social responsibility or because a healthier, more engaged workforce makes good business sense. A motivated, healthy workforce is more likely to perform well. Employers and employees benefit through improved morale, reduced absenteeism, increased retention and improved productivity.

22. There are some simple measures employers can take to promote health in the workplace. For example, Inland Revenue rules allow employers to help staff in a number of ways to increase their physical activity by cycling to work, including through tax-efficient bike purchase from salary. The use of these concessions is low, in part because of lack of knowledge and understanding. **The Department for Transport will work with the cycle industry to produce user-friendly guidance on the tax-efficient bike purchase scheme to increase the use of the scheme and promote cycling.**

Primary care trusts are also now being encouraged to be much more proactive in their management of local supply to ensure access for all. Incentives to attract new providers will be developed to ensure that everyone has fair access to primary care near their home and/or workplace.

Ref: 2.8 NHS Improvement Plan

The Department for Culture, Media and Sport (DCMS) has introduced a number of changes to help promote a healthy workplace and to get staff more active. These include: stair prompts to encourage staff to take the stairs; provision of pedometers; investment in new bike racks and shower facilities to encourage cycling to work; and healthier options in the canteen and vending machines.

Through a new partnership with the Central YMCA, the DCMS is upgrading its in-house gym equipment and negotiating a special deal for staff who want to use the Central YMCA's facilities and has introduced yoga classes to broaden the offer to existing members and encourage more to join. A running club has also been set up, giving staff the chance to get fit and socialise with colleagues at the same time. Making use of the green spaces on DCMS's doorstep, the club welcomes men and women, regardless of ability, and holds lunchtime sessions specially designed for absolute beginners.

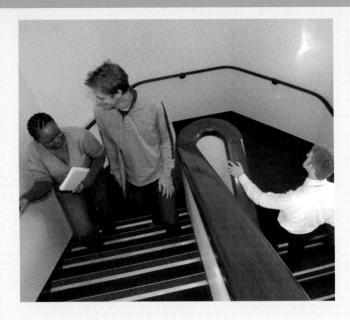

23. The NHS can also help. NHS services, such as walk-in centres, already provide easier access to health services close to work. Expansion and diversification of NHS health improvement services will ensure that they become just as convenient and accessible as healthcare services. The NHS and employers can also work in partnership to improve the health of their employees, for example through agreements with local NHS health trainers or NHS Stop Smoking Services to promote access to their services.

Promoting workplace health

24. Workplaces are often underutilised as a setting for promoting health and well-being. This is something that inidivdual employees cannot achieve for themselves but need assistance from employers, Government and trades unions. We know a good deal about ways in which job and environmental design can help promote health. And we know that providing opportunities for activity and a healthy diet, and help to give up smoking, is important. Although a review by the US Centers for Disease Control and Prevention has concluded that behaviour change programmes in the workplace can work, we need more rigorous evidence of what works in the UK.

25. We will establish pilots to develop the evidence base for effectiveness on promoting health and well-being through the workplace.[5] Each pilot will focus on a specific type of workplace, such as an NHS organisation, a local council or a business.

26. The programme will assess innovative approaches to support active living and also to promote healthy eating, smoking cessation and smoke-free environments, emotional and mental health and preventing back pain. A central focus will be on approaches that encourage self-management, personal responsibility and providing support to enable healthy choices.

Building health in

27. Employers have recognised the benefits of investing in their staff in the context of education and development, which is why the Investors in People (IiP) Standard has been so successful. Investing in health and well-being should be a key component of investment in staff. **We have agreed with IiP that they will develop a new healthy business assessment, in conjunction with DH, identifying the advantages for business and employees in investing in staff health and building on mechanisms already available to businesses from IiP covering issues such as work – life balance. This work will be incorporated into the IiP Standard when it is next reviewed in 2007.**

5   This programme is being developed in partnership with Sport England, the British Heart Foundation, Business in the Community and the Big Lottery Fund.

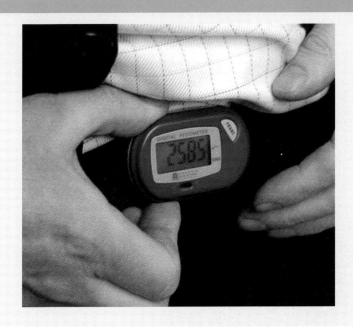

GOVERNMENT AND THE PUBLIC SECTOR: LEADING BY EXAMPLE

28. We are aware that Government and the public sector have real issues to tackle in improving the health of our workforce. Government recognises that individual employees alone cannot achieve this improvement, but need help from their public service employers. We want to learn from best practice elsewhere and find practical ways to promote the health of public sector employees, so that we lead by example as employers. For example, Sport England activity consultancy offers a flagship example of how this can be achieved.

Leading by example on smoke-free workplaces

29. **Recognising the importance of leading by example, we, as central Government, want to end all smoking in all our enclosed workplaces by 2006. We will be consulting with staff and unions on how to put this into practice.** Implementation of the ban on smoking will be supplemented by advice and support for those employees who want to stop smoking.

30. **The Health Development Agency will shortly publish guidance for NHS organisations on the provision of smoke-free buildings to protect staff, patients and others from the health risks of second-hand smoke.** In line with the wider strategy on second-hand smoke outlined in Chapter 4, NHS organisations should take action to eliminate second-hand smoke from all their buildings and provide comprehensive support for smokers who want to give up. We recognise that in some cases, such as mental hospitals where for some patients the hospital may be their main place of residence and therefore their home, this may not be achievable. The guidance will therefore provide practical advice for a wide range of settings.

31. Nurses make up the largest staff group in the NHS and their health matters, for themselves, for the NHS and for their patients. Too many nurses smoke and many of them want to stop, so we want to give them more support to stop smoking. **A joint Department of Health and Royal College of Nursing campaign will ensure that nurses are at the forefront of a smoke-free NHS by providing:**

- **personalised support for nurses wanting to stop;**
- **an award for teams that quit;**
- **a dedicated helpline for nurses;**
- **better access to nicotine replacement therapy;**
- **new self-help materials for nurses;**
- **a checklist for directors of nursing on how to help nurses to quit; and**
- **learning materials for student nurses.**

Although we are starting with nurses, this is an approach that could be adopted with other staff groups across the NHS to support health improvement at work.

CASE STUDY

The NHS has embarked on a massive recruitment programme but cannot get the staff it needs. Yet it often operates in areas of high unemployment, where poverty makes local residents more vulnerable to illness. Until now, these people have seldom been considered as candidates for health service jobs as: they lack basic skills and qualifications; they do not hear about NHS vacancies; or their knowledge and experience is undervalued or unrecognised.

There are now moves to recruit locally by investing NHS funds in pre-employment training and starting people off in jobs that require few skills, to help them move up the NHS 'skills escalator'. This provides access points at every level of training to ensure a constant stream of new recruits moving through the system. Some trusts are already adopting this approach. Such a long-term strategy is capable over time of reducing risks to health as well as developing a local workforce.

The NHS as an employer

32. The NHS makes a valuable contribution to health by providing 1.3 million jobs. But too often NHS organisations have not been model employers and do not pay sufficient attention to the health of the people who work for them. A number of studies in the NHS have shown that patient care is affected by the experience of staff: staff who have positive attitudes towards their work are more likely to work more effectively and efficiently. So paying more attention to the health of NHS staff will benefit both the NHS organisations and their patients.

33. The *NHS Plan* introduced the Improving Working Lives Standard against which over 600 NHS organisations have been assessed. Achievement of the standards is monitored by the Healthcare Commission and contributes to star ratings. Since November 2003, 13 organisations have been piloting Practice Plus, a series of higher standards demonstrating organisation-wide commitment. All NHS organisations will achieve Practice Plus status by the end of March 2006.

34. We believe that the NHS can and will become an exemplar for public and private sector employers. We will set out how the NHS will continue to develop employment policies and practices to make better, healthier NHS

workplaces in the NHS workforce strategy that we are currently developing. This will provide details of how we develop a workforce to deliver the NHS Improvement Plan and the challenges set out in this White Paper. These initiatives will be supported by workplace pilots which will, in particular, encourage staff to be more physically active.

35. To achieve this, NHS organisations will need to give careful consideration to a range of factors, including:

- the expansion of staff required to boost capacity in public health and healthcare interventions, particularly diagnostics and the management of long-term conditions;
- the expected productivity benefits from skill-mix and role-redesign;
- the levels of international recruitment needed in nursing and key specialties; and
- taking steps to support good health in a high-quality workforce representative of the population it serves.

Healthcare Commission Staff Survey

The 2003 NHS staff survey was carried out by the Healthcare Commission to provide individual NHS employers, policy-makers and national regulators with information about the attitudes and experiences of staff.

The survey conducted in October 2003 is probably the largest workforce survey in the world. Five hundred and seventy-two organisations took part, and a total of 203,911 NHS employees responded (54% of those invited).

Although three-quarters of NHS staff said they are generally satisfied with their jobs, compared with two-thirds in similar surveys of other sectors, half felt under pressure at work. In addition, over a third of staff have experienced harassment, bullying or abuse at work in the previous 12 months, mainly from patients and relatives.

36. **We will work with the NHS Employers' Organisation to ensure that the recently published *Framework for Vocational Rehabilitation*, which is the first step towards developing a new approach to helping people back to work following injury, illness or impairment, is adopted by NHS employers.**

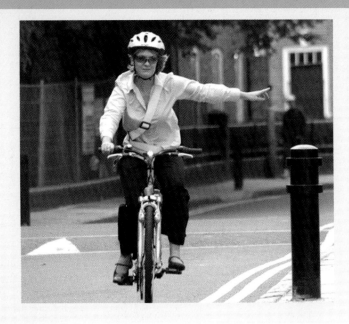

37. World-class organisations recognise the value of good people management and the importance of measuring the contribution of the workforce to providing high-quality services. We are working with SHAs to develop an HR Balanced Scorecard to help NHS organisations more effectively measure people management policies and procedures. This process will allow local NHS organisations to develop indicators that reflect the importance of staff health and well-being in creating a world-class workforce. In addition, **we will work with the Healthcare Commission and the NHS Employers' Organisation to develop the annual NHS staff survey so that we can better assess current practice and encourage more NHS organisations to become healthier workplaces.**

Improving Working Lives Standards
What are they?

A series of standards demonstrating good HR practice against which all NHS organisations have been assessed and accredited. The standards ensure that NHS employees work in an organisation that can demonstrate:

- commitment to flexible working conditions, giving staff more control over their own time;
- that they are investing in diversity and tackling discrimination and harassment; and
- that staff feel valued and treated with respect and dignity.

Why are we doing it?

So that the NHS is seen as a model employer, where individuals choose to come and work. Achieving improvements in healthcare needs a workforce able to deliver that care. Recruitment and retention of staff is key to delivering the *NHS Plan*. Given the demographic changes within the workforce, the NHS has to compete with other organisations for a limited number of people. The NHS has to be an employer that treats its staff well.

Occupational health

38. NHS organisations, as the largest employer, must also lead by example on occupational health. In the last six years up to 2002–03, support from occupational health has reduced by 50%, the number of staff forced to take ill-health retirement. **We will develop NHS occupational health services to increase the focus on quality and customer need. Altered working arrangements and the use of evidence-based practice will increase capacity and allow concentration on what the NHS needs in terms of staff and patient protection and attendance management.**

Mental health

39. Reports show that mental illness is a problem for NHS employees.

40. Improving line management skills can help improve mental well-being for staff. **The NHS Leadership Centre and NHSU support the development of leadership capability and capacity. Through national programmes, including Managing Health and Social Care, they will promote learning opportunities for leaders and managers on both wider public health issues and the responsibilities of managers to support and improve the health of staff.**

41. Building on the publication *Mental Health and Employment in the NHS*, published in 2002, **we will develop with partners[6] guidelines on the management of mild to moderate mental ill health in the workplace to be published in 2005.**

CONCLUSION

42. There are strong links between employment, individual health and the health of local communities. It is in all our interests to take forward action to support people into employment and improve opportunities for good health in the workplace. Income from employment increases the potential for people to make healthy choices; employees can benefit personally from being in a healthy workplace; for the employer, their workforce is their most important resource and society benefits from high employment and a fit and productive workforce.

6   British Occupational Health Research Foundation and the Sainsbury Centre for Mental Health and Mentality.

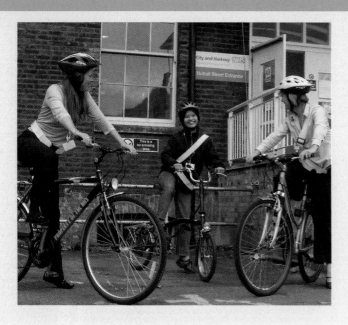

Summary

43. The initiatives described in this chapter will
ensure that there are better opportunities for
health through work and the workplace.

- More people who are currently out of the
  workforce will be employed, reducing
  inequalities in employment and health.
- The NHS will be working in partnership with
  other public sector agencies, such as Jobcentre
  Plus, and employers to help those who can
  return to work, for their own good, the good
  of their employers and of wider society.
- Workplaces will become healthier environments.
- There will be better support for employers to
  help develop the health of their workforce.
- Central Government, NHS organisations and
  other parts of the public sector will lead
  as examples of healthy employers.

SCENARIO
WHAT WILL HEALTH LOOK LIKE IN THE FUTURE?

Dan is 50. He was divorced nine years ago and moved out of the family home. He works for a company that employs 500 people, making electrical parts.

Dan has found his job difficult since his team was given a new team leader, who is constantly pushing to meet targets. He starts to sleep badly and feel tired and anxious at work. Eventually, Dan visits his GP, who signs him off work.

Dan's GP also notices that Dan has not updated his personalised health guide (PHG) since he left school and advises him to go for a 'health check' – a new service for people entering their 50s. Dan is reluctant until he discovers he can access some of the service from home, using the digital TV package he bought for watching football. He books time one evening to talk to an NHS Direct nurse, who appears live on his TV screen. She asks him about his health and lifestyle and records this information in his PHG.

The health check shows that Dan generally eats poorly and does little exercise. Dan agrees to look at some websites about healthy eating. He also agrees to try and go for a daily walk while he is off work.

After some weeks, Dan's company sends one of its occupational health consultants to see him about returning to work. It allows him to move teams

and work part-time for some weeks. It also agrees to review its policies on target setting and to provide 'break out' rooms for other employees in danger of suffering from stress. Meanwhile, Dan's PHG has been loaded onto the HealthSpace website, where he can access it using a secure password. He makes a note about what he has agreed with the company's occupational health adviser, so his GP can see it the next time his PHG is called up.

Dan also decides to have a full health check and books an appointment for one at his local surgery. The walks have helped to control his stress symptoms, so he asks the health-check technician about the health benefits of starting to run.

The two find a suitable programme on a running magazine website. This is attached to his PHG. However, Dan also decides to pay for a subscription to the magazine, so he can receive a personalised programme, training and eating tips by text.

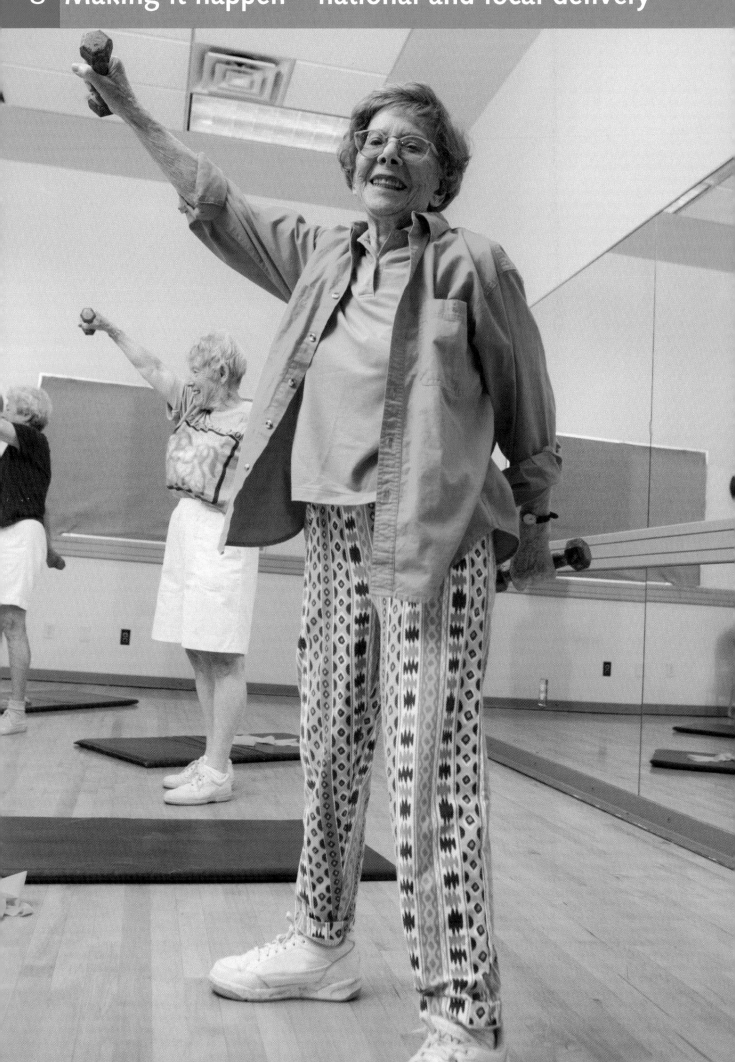

'There has been so much written [on Public Health policy] often covering similar ground and apparently sound, setting out well-known major determinants of health, but rigorous implementation of identified solutions has often been sadly lacking.'

Derek Wanless, February 2004

INTRODUCTION

1. The Government is determined that this White Paper should make a difference to people's lives. Turning its commitments into sustained action will be everybody's business

2. This chapter sets out the key actions by which national government should be judged:

- regulation;
- resourcing delivery;
- joining up action;
- aligning planning and performance assessment;
- building partnerships and inviting engagement.

It also summarises how action will be ensured locally, particularly through local government and the NHS. Annex B has a more detailed description of those delivery mechanisms and how they will be used. The Annex also outlines how we will get sufficient workforce capacity and capability to deliver.

3. To avoid the risk that in some cases, interventions may contribute to widening health inequalities, government departments, and particularly the Office of the Deputy Prime Minister and Department of Health, will ensure that initiatives and programmes are health inequality 'proofed'. This will involve consideration of whether any policy changes or remedial actions are necessary to prevent any negative effects on health

inequalities. The impact of 'non-health' interventions on population health should also be more routinely considered both before implementing policies (through Health Impact Assessments, for example) and afterwards through evaluation.

REGULATION

4. **The Government will build health into all future legislation by including health as a component in regulatory impact assessment.**

5. The Government will take responsibility for ensuring detailed consultation on proposals to legislate in this White Paper, with the aim of bringing forward promptly the policies set out to regulate smoking in public places and workplaces, on the standard of food provided in schools over the whole school day and to tighten regulation of underage tobacco sales.

6. The Government will continue to take tough action on tobacco smuggling. Over the past two decades, establishing and maintaining a high level of tax on cigarettes – as has been the policy of successive governments – has been shown to help reduce smoking prevalence. Cigarette duty was subject to a sustained period of real-terms increases during the 1990s, and has been held at the present high level in real terms since 2000–01. Compared to many other countries, the UK has high duties on tobacco products and high-priced cigarettes.

However, an increase in the availability of cheaper, illegally smuggled cigarettes and hand-rolling tobacco has meant that some smokers have been able to by-pass higher prices, undermining the impact of price on smoking prevalence rates and meaning that further real increases in duty would be likely to be of limited effectiveness.

7. Tobacco smuggling undermines the Government's tobacco control strategy, as well as stimulating serious widespread criminality. Smuggling brings in large volumes of cheap cigarettes – including counterfeit cigarettes – making smoking more accessible to young people and those on low incomes. Major inroads have been made in the last few years to tackle the problem and Customs have succeeded in slowing, stabilising and reversing the growth in cigarette smuggling. **We have reduced the smuggled share of the cigarette market to 18% in 2002–03, and aim to reduce this further to no more than 13% by 2007–08.**

8. The question of how best to regulate tobacco products was an issue raised in the Wanless report and in the public consultation on *Choosing Health?* Although we do not think that there is a case for setting up a brand new UK agency to regulate tobacco, as some have called for, we recognise the need for more work to look at how best to regulate tobacco products. We are in discussion with the European Commission and working with partner agencies, including Medicine and Healthcare products Regulatory Agency (MHRA) who regulate medicinal nicotine products such as nicotine patches and gum for quitting, the Health Protection Agency (HPA), our expert scientific advisory committees and the National Institute for Clinical Excellence (NICE),[1] to develop a strategy for taking this work forward. In 2005 we expect to see a report from the European Commission which will give a view of the cross-Europe priorities for work in this area.

RESOURCING DELIVERY

9. Some of the initiatives to improve health in this White Paper will rely on focusing mainstream programmes and innovative service design on public health objectives. Others will entail extra costs. Most are the responsibility of the Department of Health. The Secretary of State for Health has committed to provide the new funding identified against specific proposals. This includes new money for stimulating demand for health through campaigns, more school nurses, the introduction of health trainers and better obesity and sexual health services.

10. We will give funding priority to areas of greatest need, to address health inequalities. This will provide more flexibility for local partners, including local

1   See Annex B for detail on the further development of NICE's role in public health.

authorites, to decide on how best to resource local activities through, for example, more efficient working arrangements or more effective targeting of services to reduce overall demand.

JOINED-UP ACTION

11. The Government is committed to the New Burdens Doctrine and will reimburse local authorities fully for any extra costs they face as a result of the policies in this White Paper. We will be working with local government to assess the resource implications of relevant initiatives before they are implemented.

12. To ensure Government itself demonstrates the joined up action that it asks of others, the Secretary of State for Health will coordinate action through the new Cabinet Sub Committee, set up to oversee the development and implementation of the Government's policies to improve public health and reduce health inequalities.

13. The Government will also pursue its approach to choosing health internationally, and has adopted 'Empowering people, reducing inequalities', as one of its themes for the UK's EU Presidency in the second half of 2005.

14. Last year's cross-government Health Inequalities Programme for Action identified four key areas for progress:

- supporting families, mothers and children;
- engaging communities and individuals;
- preventing illness and providing effective treatment and care; and
- addressing the underlying determinants of health.

15. We will publish a follow-up report on progress against the strategy. This will look at the national health inequalities target on life expectancy and infant mortality, together with progress against the 12 national health inequalities indicators and on the delivery of commitments by government departments set out in the Programme for Action.

16. This White Paper now makes specific commitments in each of the key areas, to focus effort over the next period. This is by no means the end of the story. Experience of service improvement in the NHS and elsewhere suggests that by focusing on a small number of priorities at the outset delivery is secured and momentum built for sustained change.

17. The White Paper also demonstrates how we are putting joined up action into practice to improve health. There will also be specific joint programmes of action on those targets/goals to which departments have already made joint commitments. These include:

- halting the year-on-year rise in obesity among children under 11 by 2010 in the context of a broader strategy to tackle obesity in the population as a whole. Joint target between the Department of Health, the Department for Education and Skills (DfES) and the Department of Culture, Media and Sport; and
- reducing the under-18 conception rate by 50% by 2010, as part of a broader strategy to improve sexual health. Joint target between the Department of Health and the DfES.

18. To ensure public accountability and demonstrate continuing progress the Department of Health will publish a six monthly progress report on key indicators for the targets that relate directly to improving health. These reports will reflect the joint contributions of all departments involved.

NATIONAL PLANS FOR DELIVERY

19. The Government will publish a Delivery Plan for the White Paper early next year. This will make clear the accountability for the commitments we have made and the action that needs to be taken. It will spell out the particular roles and responsibilities for health improvement of all health and social care organisations and, where we have reached agreements, for organisations in the rest of the public, private and voluntary sectors.

20. As part of this delivery programme we will also – as previously promised – publish discrete national delivery plans focusing on nutrition and activity, including:

- the Food and Health Action Plan;
- the Physical Activity Plan.

These will set out how and when Government, its agencies and others will deliver their commitments to improve the nation's diet and increase activity, including those commitments identified in this White Paper and other relevant Departmental plans.[2] In particular, the Food and Health Action Plan will coordinate with, and contribute to the delivery of, the *Strategy for Sustainable Farming and Food* (SSFF). As part of that we will ensure that the regional delivery plans of the SSFF all include commitments on nutrition. The plans will help coordinate the work of national, regional and local government, the voluntary sector, business and others. Together with other parts of the White Paper delivery plan, the plans will show how we will deliver the cross-Government public service agreement on halting the year-on-year rise in obesity in children.

21. Individual Government departments will also be publishing their own five-year delivery plans in the coming months. These include the Office of the Deputy Prime Minister, the Department for

---

2   For example, Department for Transport, *Walking and Cycling: An Action Plan*, launched June 2004.

'(The ingredients of success are) effective performance management, clear priorities, targets, good real time data, management against trajectory and the capacity to intervene where necessary'.

Michael Barber, Prime Minister's Delivery Unit

Culture Media and Sport and the Department for Environment, Food and Rural Affairs, whose plans will be relevant to the implementation of this White Paper.

BUILDING PARTNERSHIPS AND INVITING ENGAGEMENT FOR DELIVERY

22. Development work as well as direct action is needed to take forward the ideas in this White Paper. We shall work on this with local government, the NHS, consumer and voluntary organisations and the private sector.

23. We will organise the first national conference within a month of publication to allow as many key players as possible to engage with our approach supporting healthy choices. This will lead into a series of regional roadshows to present the main messages in this White Paper and to encourage commitment from around the country.

24. To encourage organisations to make their pledges to improve health, described in Chapter 4, we will ensure that within six months there is a mechanism for everyone to record their pledges publicly. The first awards to celebrate achievements in improving health will be made in 2005. We will encourage individuals with the right skills and enthusiasm to join a network of health champions, to help organisations which want to improve health.

ENSURING ACTION LOCALLY: A CLEAR SYSTEM FOR DELIVERY

25. In order to achieve the step change needed in health improvement we need to make most effective use of the developing structural and organisational frameworks involving NHS bodies, local authorities, and the business, voluntary and community sectors. These include the creation of integrated statutory organisations such as Care Trusts, and partnership arrangements through children's trusts, and on a broader level Local Strategic Partnerships. Local leadership and commitment is vital and these partnerships provide an important forum for elected and board-level members, Chief Executives and other senior representatives to develop a shared vision and agenda for action to improve health.

26. Our approach for local delivery of improved health by the NHS and local government will be based on central government aligning for local partners. It will consist of:

- standards for services;
- targets, which are increasingly based on outcomes;
- incentives;
- support for change; and
- inspection and performance assessment.

'Healthcare organisations in the past have tended to focus on ill-health. The Healthcare Commission's systems of assessment will look at the contribution that healthcare organisations are making to improve the health and well-being of the population as well as reducing inequalities in the standard of health enjoyed by different sections of our community. By working in partnership with a broad range of inspectorates we will play a key role in improving public health.'

Sir Ian Kennedy, Chairman of the Healthcare Commission

27. From 2005, we are introducing a new performance framework for all health and social care organisations, *Standards for Better Health*. One of the areas it covers is public health. The standards will form a key part of the Healthcare Commission's assessment of all healthcare organisations.

28. The White Paper reinforces the importance of the Public Service Agreement targets which have already been set to improve health and reduce inequalities. Delivery of these targets will be primarily through the work of the NHS and local government. For the NHS, improving health has also been identified as one of the four national priorities for the period to 2008, putting health goals alongside service delivery as a top priority for every NHS organisation, every NHS Chair and every Chief Executive. In local government, tackling health inequalities is one of the shared priorities endorsed by the Local Government Association.

29. There is a range of incentives available to encourage progress towards the White Paper objectives and empower partners to work more effectively. In local government, councils can receive extra government funding for achieving more ambitious local targets, such as those on tackling health inequalities. The introduction of Local Area Agreements offers significant

opportunities for PCTs, councils and other partners to address improvements in the health of their communities. In the NHS, the Local Delivery Planning process focuses management attention on key targets and acts as a driver for step changes in performance. To reinforce this, it would be possible to encourage the development of new services by making the release of funding conditional on evidence of a robust, specific plan which addresses both capacity and capability and outlines clear delivery mechanisms. The local delivery plan process will engage all of the relevant local partners, including councils, in addressing public health priorities. Taken together with Local Area Agreements this process should support development of a shared agenda for all relevant partners and provide greater flexibility to achieve agreed priorities.

30. Supporting implementation of the White Paper proposals in the NHS and local government will be a priority task for the Modernisation Agency (and its replacement body), the Improvement and Development Agency and the Care Service Improvement Partnership. Funding will be available to support transformational change on the ground. Both agencies will work together to provide health improvement expertise, best practice tools and ideas on how to encourage local areas to adopt them rapidly. In time, extra support will be made

available to organisations which fail to make satisfactory progress on health improvement.

31. We will also publish revised Health and Neighbourhood Renewal Guidance in 2005, which will highlight good practice for organisations working together in Local Strategic Partnerships.

32. The Healthcare Commission and Audit Commission have agreed to work together to find ways to align their new performance systems for assessing health improvement and reduction in health inequalities.

33. They will also develop a framework for improvement reviews of public health issues as well as jointly reviewing and developing data sets on public health.

34. These actions will ensure that health is core business for the NHS and local government and their partners, and part of mainstream systems for incentives, performance, regulation and inspection which are aligned to support community development, health improvement service delivery and individual behavioural change.

CONCLUSION

35. Meeting the new health challenges of the 21st century will need a step change in action. These arrangements reflect the need for Government, communities and individuals to take seriously their respective responsibilities for health. The commitments in this White Paper are designed to ensure more healthy choices are available and to shape the environment so that these choices are readily available to those who would otherwise be disadvantaged. This is the beginning of a journey to build health into Government policy and ensure that health is everybody's business. This chapter shows the Government is serious about ensuring that these commitments are met and that this time we get sustained and focused action to improve people's health.

ANNEX A
CHOOSING HEALTH? CONSULTATION

INTRODUCTION

In preparation for this White Paper, the Department of Health (DH) launched the *Choosing Health?* consultation on 3 March 2004. This ran until 28 June 2004. In parallel with the *Choosing Health?* consultation, the DH also carried out two separate consultations on physical activity and diet through the Choosing Activity and Choosing a Better Diet consultations respectively.

The consultation was held to generate ideas and indicate the concerns of a wide range of stakeholders, including: individuals, public organisations, private organisations, charitable and non-governmental organisations and communities, which would then feed into the formulation of the White Paper.

The consultation aimed to engage as many people and partners as possible in discussion on how best to improve health, with a range of activities undertaken in support of the consultation, including:

- local consultation events led by primary care trusts (PCTs) and local authorities;

- regional consultation led by Regional Directors of Public Health;

- national consultation led by task groups involving 200 experts focusing on eight identified themes:

  - better health for children and young people;

  - working for health/opportunities in employment;

  - consumers and markets;

  - leisure;

- maximising the NHS contribution – in primary care;

- maximising the NHS contribution – across the NHS as a whole;

- working with and for communities; and

- focusing on delivery.

■ national summits on tackling inequalities and dealing with the challenges of poor diet and inactivity;

■ focused events, such as for people in black and minority ethnic communities, on improving mental wellbeing and encouraging health improvement for people with chronic mental illness;

■ an independent omnibus survey of public opinion on what it is important for the Government to do, and what the priorities are, to improve health;

■ DH Ministers have held four breakfast seminars with 62 senior representatives from key public sector organisations; and

■ the King's Fund hosted two seminars on the role of the media and the role of government in public health.

An overview of the responses to the consultation is set out below. Some information from the independent survey has already been published and is available from Opinion Leader Research (www.kingsfund/pdf/publicattitudesreport.pdf). A fuller analysis of the consultations, further information from the survey and the recommendations of the chairs of the eight task groups will be made available on the DH website (www.dh.gov.uk).

RESPONSES

2,230 submissions were received (by post or e-mail) to the *Choosing Health?* consultation. In addition, 283 responses were received to the Choosing Activity consultation and 218 responses were received from the Choosing a Better Diet consultation. The collection of information and forms of consultation that were held to inform these submissions was varied, ranging from focus groups with specific user groups, communities and localities to large-scale questionnaires given out in both healthcare and non-healthcare settings. Over 153,000 individuals were involved in total in the consultation.

A wide range of organisations and individuals responded to the *Choosing Health?* consultation, with very high numbers of responses from individuals (1,080), PCTs (325) and non-governmental and charitable organisations (204). The number of responses from other organisations was also high for a public consultation; 93 responses were received from business and industry and 141 were received from local government. There was also a wide geographical spread. A wide range of respondent types also contributed to the Choosing Activity and Choosing a Better Diet consultations.

CHOOSING HEALTH? CONSULTATION RESULTS

The main subject areas covered by submissions to the *Choosing Health?* consultation were:

- smoking;
- diet and nutrition;
- physical activity; and
- the NHS contribution.

The main proposals for action emerging in these and other areas from the consultation are set out in the table below.

Cross-cutting themes

Following analysis of the responses to consultation, certain themes were evident in the responses covering the subject areas listed above. These were the importance of work with children, the role of work and the workplace, the need to develop skills and information for health and the need for joined-up thinking and action.

Results of consultation analysis for *Choosing Health?*	
Subject area	**Main issues raised**
Smoking	Restrictions in workplaces/public places.
Diet and nutrition	Advertising/labelling, particularly: ■ restrictions on advertising food to children; and ■ more information and simple nutrition messages on food.
Physical activity	Access to leisure centres/facilities for physical activity, particularly: ■ reducing barriers such as costs, travel and lack of childcare; and ■ lack of information about local facilities.
NHS contribution	Concentration on prevention of ill-health.
Health inequalities	Targeted work with high-risk groups.
Mental health	Action to tackle stress, particularly: ■ in the work context; and ■ young people's emotional well-being.
Alcohol misuse	Tackling anti-social behaviour.
Sexually transmitted infections	More information/public education.
Accidents	Road safety/accidents.
Drug misuse	Information provision, particularly clearer messages focused on young people.
Wider determinants of health	Need for action on wider determinants with a particular focus on transport and children's education.

CHOOSING ACTIVITY CONSULTATION RESULTS

The main proposals for action emerging in the Choosing Activity consultation were to:

- improve information and raise awareness of the benefits of activity;

- support activity in the community by addressing barriers such as safety, cost, and locality;

- support activity in early years and schools and improve community access to school facilities; and

- support and encourage everyday activity such as walking and cycling.

CHOOSING A BETTER DIET CONSULTATION RESULTS

The main proposals for action emerging in the Choosing a Better Diet consultation were:

- improving information and education on food issues, including better food labelling;

- improving diet for children and young people, especially in schools;

- improving the range of healthier foods, eg producing food with less fat, sugar and salt content;

- helping communities to help themselves, eg through improved access to healthy foods; and

- increasing support from the NHS.

CONCLUSION

Engagement in the *Choosing Health?* consultation was extremely high, and the level of submissions alone indicates the importance many organisations and individuals attach to the subjects concerned. Overall, the consultation clearly illustrated the exceptional level of interest that currently exists in improving health and reflected a very strong will for action on major policy issues.

ANNEX B
MAKING IT HAPPEN

1. The key to national health improvement is more people making
    healthier choices more of the time. Many of the proposals in this
    White Paper will help make the healthy choice the easy choice for
    people. Other proposals will develop an environment where
    people who are disadvantaged in making those healthy choices
    will increasingly have similar opportunities to others.

2. This annex sets out how we will ensure that there is a strong system to deliver
    everywhere the commitments we make in this White Paper, and how can we build
    on the popular support for action to create irreversible momentum for change.
    To do this we propose actions in three broad areas:

    ▪ Evidence and Information

    ▪ Workforce Capacity and Capability

    ▪ Systems for Local Delivery

3. The diagram below sets out the relationship between these three areas:

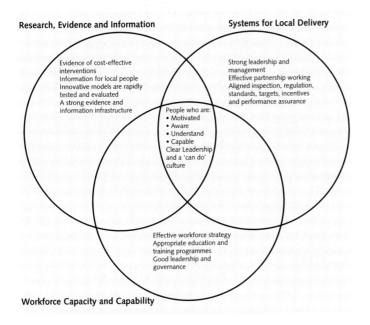

Research, Evidence and Information

Evidence of cost-effective interventions
Information for local people
Innovative models are rapidly tested and evaluated
A strong evidence and information infrastructure

Systems for Local Delivery

Strong leadership and management
Effective partnership working
Aligned inspection, regulation, standards, targets, incentives and performance assurance

People who are:
• Motivated
• Aware
• Understand
• Capable
Clear Leadership and a 'can do' culture

Effective workforce strategy
Appropriate education and training programmes
Good leadership and governance

Workforce Capacity and Capability

4. We will publish a delivery plan in early 2005 which will give more detail on how we will implement each of the commitments we have made in the White Paper. This will build on relevant activity already in hand. So, for example, we will ensure that activities relevant to children and young people are brought together with work underway to improve children's health under the 'be healthy' strand of *Every child matters: delivering change for children*.

EVIDENCE AND INFORMATION FOR ACTION
The challenge

5. In 'Securing Good Health for the Whole Population', Derek Wanless was critical of the dearth of evidence available on what works in health improvement. He called for action to strengthen the evidence base on interventions and their cost-effectiveness, for improved use of information on the population and its health status, and for a sharper focus on using evidence and information to inform practice. He also called for evaluation of new initiatives as a rapid means of filling gaps in the evidence base.

Action to strengthen public health research

6. Action on improving health has been hampered by gaps in the evidence on what works best to support and sustain change in people's behaviour, and how to do this most cost-effectively.

'Although there is often evidence on the scientific justification for action and for some specific interventions, there is generally little evidence about the cost-effectiveness of public health and preventative policies or their practical implication. Research in this area can be technically difficult and there is a lack of depth and expertise in the core disciplines. This, coupled with a lack of funding of public health intervention research and slower acceptance of economic perspectives within public health, all contribute to the dearth of evidence of cost-effectiveness.'
Derek Wanless, February 2004

7. The key challenges we need to address are:

■ research funding and effort has not met the needs of front line staff for good evidence on what will improve the public's health;

■ lack of an overarching national strategy for public health has resulted in failure to systematically identify the research gaps and prioritise commissioning of research to fill these;

■ insufficient co-ordination between the different research funders and between the researchers and those charged with front line actions to improve health;

■ lack of funding for research into the interventions that will support and sustain behaviour change, and those which will tackle health inequalities;

■ too long a time lag between conception of a new idea and getting it into practice;

■ a lack of research capacity with the mix of skills and expertise needed, good links between the

NHS and academia and clear career pathways; there are important areas of strength, like epidemiology, but expertise in areas including promoting behaviour change is more limited; and

■ there is limited evidence on cost-effectiveness.

8. **We will review the existing R&D strategy for public health to provide a strategy focused on supporting delivery of this White Paper through improved, timely, evidence.**

9. To meet the challenges this will set, **we will establish a new public health research initiative within the framework of the United Kingdom Clinical Research Collaboration (UKCRC).** This will bring together research funding partners, including the Research Councils and the Wellcome Trust, to agree the long-term research strategy. This co-ordinated approach will make the necessary connections across Government, with the National Institute for Clinical Excellence and with the wider public health information community and consumer interests. It will benefit from working closely with UKCRC workstreams on the research workforce and the regulatory and governance environment.

10. **Starting in 2005–06, the Government will provide new funding for the public health research initiative, building to £10m by 2007–08.** This is on top of existing plans to increase spend by the Department of Health Policy Research Programme on public health research to £10m per annum by 2006.

11. **Following the White Paper, we will make an early start by launching two projects to strengthen the evidence base on work to improve health. Early in 2005, we will launch a public health research consortium, bringing together national policy makers and researchers from a wide range of disciplines relevant to public health, to focus effort on strengthening the evidence for effective health interventions to support White Paper delivery.**

12. **We shall launch a National Prevention Research Initiative, working in collaboration with research funders in the fields of obesity, cancer, coronary heart disease and diabetes, to provide dedicated funding for research aimed at the primary prevention of these diseases.** This will build on existing work between DH and partners through the National Cancer Research Institute. The emphasis will be on studies on the development, evaluation and implementation of interventions to influence behaviour. This includes research aimed at reducing smoking, improving diet and nutrition, preventing obesity and increasing physical activity.

13. Action to build the public health workforce will include steps to strengthen the academic infrastructure, to build closer links between field practitioners and academic centres, and to strengthen the research and evaluation skills of all public health practitioners.

Action on evidence of cost effectiveness and best practice

14. To complement these new developments on research, we shall act to strengthen evidence of cost effectiveness, and to make evidence of what works more readily available to inform and develop frontline practice and to capture evidence of what works from new models of practice in the field.

15. In July 2004, as part of the Department of Health's wider review of Arms Length Bodies, we announced our plans to transfer the functions of the Health Development Agency (HDA) to the National Institute for Clinical Excellence (NICE), to form a new body with a wider focus on both care and health, and create a Centre for Public Health Excellence. This will build on the complementary experience and skills of the two organisations, with their track records of successful delivery. It will bring to bear the rigour of economic appraisal, which NICE has developed in its work on clinical topics in the NHS, on the wider public health

evidence base already gathered by the HDA, and on future evidence. And it will develop and strengthen the regional presence of the HDA, to ensure that frontline practice is shaped and developed in line with the evidence base.

16. The challenge for both bodies is to create a strong, new organisation which will be called the National Institute for Health & Clinical Excellence. This will have a broader and more complex role than either existing body. So we shall take special steps to support its development but ensure that the internationally recognised brand of NICE is retained.

17. **We will provide additional resources to support the National Institute for Health & Clinical Excellence, in its new work on health improvement.** Over and above the efficiency savings we will make from bringing HDA together with NICE, we will provide additional resources from 2006/07 to deliver specific objectives related to the White Paper.

18. **The National Institute for Health & Clinical Excellence will appoint an Executive Director for Health Improvement to provide professional leadership in delivering public health for its work across the NHS and partner organisations in local government, in education, in voluntary and community organisations. Additional Non Executive Board Members will also be appointed to improve its capacity to discharge its significantly extended role across this wider range of sectors including Local Government.**

19. For the first time, the National Institute for Health & Clinical Excellence will integrate upstream (prevention) and downstream (treatment) knowledge and guidance on effective practice and intervention as NICE and the HDA are already doing together on obesity, identifying which actions will have the greatest impact on health. It will become possible to compare evidence for the

cost effectiveness of early ill health prevention programmes with the evidence of the cost effectiveness of treatment later. The NHS and its partner organisations, including local government, will benefit from this stronger evidence base both as to what works within the field of public health, inequalities and ill-health prevention and on the case for investment upstream.

20. Bringing the experience and expertise of these two organisations together will also strengthen our ability to get evidence into practice and evaluate new interventions rapidly. We will retain and build on NICE as a strong brand with the NHS and the HDA's wider networks with other government departments and NHS partner organisations at national and at regional level, to build an internationally recognised organisation promoting excellence in public health.

Action on information

21. Good, relevant, timely information is needed to identify health problems early, to help decide what to do, and how to do it and to track progress. Information is also essential to make the case for change and investment in health.

22. Derek Wanless was surprised to observe that despite 50 years of the National Health Service,

    'Little comprehensive information is collected on the health status of the population, the prevalence of important behavioural factors, such as smoking, drinking, diet and exercise, or what the NHS actually spends its money on in relation to public health.'

    And he identified the same weaknesses at local level:

    '… there is no regular mechanism by which a PCT or local authority can gather reliable information on its own population …'

23. Some important building blocks are in place, but they do not yet add up to a coherent information system geared to today's needs. *Saving Lives: Our Healthier Nation* established Public Health Observatories in each region to support local bodies by helping them to identify local health problems and track progress in tackling them. We need now to build on their work to establish a modern public health information and intelligence system to understand the present and to model the future.

24. **Following the White Paper, we will establish a Health Information and Intelligence Task Force to lead action to develop and implement a comprehensive public health information and intelligence strategy.** Priorities for this will be to:

- develop real-time public health information leading to action at a local level, across the NHS and in the local community;

- identify an agreed set of core data, where possible from existing data sources, to support agreed measures of progress to be used nationally and locally;

- tackle weaknesses within existing data, eg information on ethnicity and use of NHS services;

- bringing together sources of information on health and wellbeing from routine sources and local studies to give a comprehensive picture of how lifestyle factors affect health;

- build on the work of Public Health Observatories on regional public health indicators to establish a framework for health surveillance at a regional level which supports a more robust national framework;

- work with the Health Protection Agency to develop effective systems, eg for sexual health;

- use new sources, such as marketing information and systems of information to improve the health of the population, including the NHS National Programme for IT, the new contract for General Medical Services and the UK Biobank;

- give guidance on data sharing, and on disclosure and confidentiality. We need to ensure that recent developments in data protection and other legislation on information are clear, and organisations are aware of what they can and can't do; and

- build on existing knowledge management systems, including the National Electronic Library for Health, to ensure information is readily available to promote best practice.

25. We will invest £5 million in 2005 and £10 million per annum from 2006 in Public Health Observatories and in developing the national public health information and intelligence strategy. This will ensure that the Public Health Observatories are better placed to support directors of public health and their teams with information and skills to promote local action and monitor its impact on health.

26. Collecting and analysing information is only half the task. Ensuring that the right people know what that information contains and understand how to use it is part of the challenge we face. For local government the Improvement and Development Agency has agreed to support the dissemination of information on approaches that demonstrate successful outcomes. Public health practitioners and NHS staff will be supported in developing skills to assist effective dissemination. Public Health Observatories will support the development of skills for example in equity audits and health impact assessments.

27. The Department will continue to work with the NHS and others on better ways of using information to inform local communities and drive

action. Chapter 4 described the new forms of local reports that Primary Care Trusts will publish to provide accessible information on the health of the local community, clearly communicated in an approachable style. Public Health Observatories will produce the information for these.

28. We are also launching a Health Poverty Index, to provide summary key information on differences in health outcomes between different areas and groups for local decision-makers. In the longer term the Government is working with the Audit Commission, Healthcare Commission and others to build in a strong health component to 'Local Area Profiles'. This will produce profiles of the quality of life and services in a local area by bringing together existing data collections.

Promoting Innovation and Evaluation Fund

29. Our new arrangements to fill gaps in the research and evidence base will take time to deliver results. Derek Wanless commented,

'...the need for action is too pressing for the lack of a comprehensive evidence base to be used as an excuse for inertia'.

He proposed a more systematic approach to the evaluation of current public health policy and practice, and of new initiatives, to identify what works, so that successful approaches can be rolled out rapidly, and those which are unsuccessful discontinued.

30. The NHS Modernisation Agency will develop a 'spread and adoption' strategy aimed to shorten the process and timescales for getting the best ideas widely taken up across local communities and organisations.

31. **We will establish a new Innovations Fund, of £30m in 2006–07 and £40m per annum from 2007–08. This will support and test new models of working and provide real-time evaluation and feedback to enable faster learning so that proven**

models can be put into practice much more rapidly than in the past.

Summary

32. This concerted drive to improve the base of information and intelligence will ensure we can meet Derek Wanless' challenge to build local and national understanding of the factors that impact on people's health at present and in future.

33. The changes set out above will mean that:

- there is a growing body of research evidence on cost-effective interventions to improve health and this informs commissioning and the practice of front line staff

- local communities see regular information about their health, trends over time, comparisons with other areas to promote local action

- innovative models of practice are tested and evaluated rapidly so that if they are successful they can be adopted as mainstream practice

- the drive for health improvement is supported by a strong infrastructure with the evidence and information systems to sustain progress.

CAPACITY AND CAPABILITY: BUILDING THE WORKFORCE
The challenge

34. The changes set out in the White Paper will only occur if the right people, with the right skills, are in place to deliver them and if barriers to change and old style professional boundaries are broken down. This means people with the right skills at all levels:

- across the wider workforce;

- as public health practitioners;

- as public health specialists; and

- in the leadership of organisations

working in a multidisciplinary workforce to respond to current problems, identify future health threats, provide expert advice and co-ordination in the delivery of high quality health improvement services and evaluate the impact of their efforts, particularly on reducing health inequalities.

The strategy

35. The NHS has already developed capacity plans to support faster access to treatment. Every national service framework – for example to improve services for people with heart disease or with mental health problems – has been supported by action to ensure the right workforce, with the right skills, is in place. This same systematic and determined approach to workforce planning and development must now be extended to health improvement. Plans will need to be aligned with mainstream NHS programmes including Agenda for Change and Modernising Medical Careers. These plans must cover not just the NHS, but also the needs of local government, voluntary organisations, academic research, and others with roles in health improvement.

36. Our overall strategy is to develop and build capacity for health improvement at all levels of the system, with the backing of a national competency framework for health to support the development of the necessary education and skills. We will identify and tackle capacity and capability gaps. Priorities will be to

   ▪ engage people from local communities in a new role as NHS health trainers, and assist them to acquire the skills to change behaviours;

   ▪ use the health trainer's development programme to accredit existing community workers or volunteers as health trainers, thereby promoting the development of skills within communities;

   ▪ better equip the wider workforce to deliver improved health by ensuring basic skills and

knowledge for more people including all those working in the NHS, by increasing understanding of key messages and how to communicate them to support behaviour change;

   ▪ ensure public health practitioners have the correct skills for their work in improving health and are used effectively;

   ▪ address critical shortfalls in specific staff groups;

   ▪ support the development of effective specialist public health practice and leadership;

   ▪ develop models for managing health improvement programmes; and

   ▪ ensure strong leadership for health improvement across organisations.

37. All staff need to be supported to understand and value their own health, and to understand and communicate the key health messages, the evidence that lies behind them and, most importantly, the most effective methods of supporting people to adopt healthy behaviours. The NHS should become as professional in its approach to delivering consistent, high quality advice and support for health as it has been traditionally in delivering high quality treatment and care. The Government are working with Skills for Health and other key stakeholders to ensure that Occupational Standards and the NHS Knowledge and Skills Framework properly reflect health improvement and the science of behaviour change.

38. **The new induction programme for all NHS staff will include basic information. In addition the curricula for pre-registration training, post-graduate education and continuous professional development will be reviewed. Staff from other local partners, particularly local authorities, including environmental health officers may also benefit from access to similar training and development. Flexible modular approaches, consistent with the NHS skills escalator will be**

developed, to create opportunities for multisectoral and lifelong learning.

Skills in the community

39. Chapter 5 describes a new role for NHS health trainers. These will be people drawn from local communities (broadly equivalent to the existing health care assistant role) who receive accredited training in health improvement, communication skills and promoting behaviour change. They will be equipped to work with people who want personal support to improve their health. **We will commission work on the core competencies for this role, as a basis for commissioning and accrediting training.** In the NHS, this will offer a first entry point to the 'skills escalator', as a potential start to a career, either in health improvement or in other areas of NHS work.

40. **We will work with the Improvement and Development Agency, the NHS Employers Organisation and other Government Departments, to establish the best way of offering elements of this training to other frontline staff – for example, housing officers, home care staff, non-teaching assistants, and staff working in leisure centres. We will explore with the relevant educational awarding bodies the possibility of developing a core curriculum for a new national Health Trainer Certificate.**

41. Since there are a number of existing models for community engagement in health improvement we propose to work initially with the 20% of PCTs with the worst health and deprivation indicators and their partners to evaluate the best ways to maximise the potential of this approach and to roll these out across the country.

42. Development of these skills and competencies will be part of the national competency framework for health. As part of this at a local level we will ensure the development of capacity and skills to deliver local initiatives, including Healthy Start,

home visiting, and sexual health information services for young people. We will ensure that capacity is developed to engage with our initiatives such as Communities for Health and to deliver the specialist competencies around obesity prevention and treatment, with particular awareness of the needs of ethnic minorities and vulnerable groups

43. We will ensure that the increased capacity needs of the services we propose, for example sexual health and occupational health, are assessed through SHAs working with their PCTs and local hospital trusts and other local partners.

Skills development for public health practitioners

44. Staff who have specific roles and skills in health improvement will have additional needs for training and skills development. These will include staff who work within a health improvement service like smoking cessation or nutrition advice; public health practitioners – including health visitors, midwives and school nurses; community pharmacists; community dentists; members of the primary care teams including GPs and other practitioners with a special interest. Others may work in the local authority workforce, such as environmental health officers and trading standards officers. Local public sector employers will need to review the numbers of people and the types of skills they need to meet the health challenges they now face and to plan for the development of these groups. Expansion of school nursing to meet the challenges set out in Chapter 3 will be a particular priority, as will health trainers.

45. There are other important groups of staff who are particularly well placed to contribute to health improvement as part of their everyday clinical practice. For example, the Pharmaceutical Public Health Strategy to be published in 2005 will discuss how best to equip pharmacists to make the most of this role.

46. There is also scope to increase engagement of staff through the new contractual arrangements as well as increasing practitioners with a special interest among GPs, nurses, midwives, health visitors and allied health professionals. **We will commission guidelines to help PCTs develop roles for practitioners with a special interest to promote health improvement.**

Increasing capacity and developing skills in public health specialists

47. Action to expand specialist capacity in public health includes:

   - expanding the number of public health specialist training posts;

   - increasing the number of healthcare graduates with experience of public health by strengthening public health input to the undergraduate curriculum;

   - offering new career pathways, for example for doctors in training through the work of Modernising Medical Careers and the Postgraduate Medical Education Training Board, and for nurses by utilising Agenda for Change;

   - improving retention of specialists in public health by creating greater flexibility in care pathways including opportunities to move between defined areas of specialist and generalist practice;

   - work with other national agencies, such as the HPA, to develop workforce capacity;

   - assess the need to develop new areas of specialist practice, such as public health genetics;

   - recruiting managers to support delivery of health improvement services;

   - exploring international recruitment and fellowships as means to developing additional specialist capacity;

   - recruiting managers to support delivery of health improvement; and

   - supporting the development of academic public health, including joint appointments with the NHS to reflect local population and delivery needs.

48. Public health specialists, including those charged with leading and delivering key health improvement services, will need to be competent to work with communities and tackle health inequalities. In addition to skills in the use of research, evaluation and information they will need skills in communications and marketing. These specialists will have an important role in training and developing other staff, to raise the skills and knowledge base of the whole workforce and ensure effective front-line delivery of services to people. Specialist training is now available for a diverse workforce from a wide range of backgrounds, all of whom need to achieve common recognised and validated standards of professional practice. **We will work with key stakeholders to ensure that training, continuing professional development and professional regulation promote the generic skills that all public health specialists will need. We will also work with stakeholders to address critical shortfalls in staff numbers.**

Leadership for health

49. Local authorities lead action on community well being. All NHS organisations will also need to provide leadership for health if the NHS is to live out the commitments to health improvement which form part of its founding purpose. Strategic leadership for health within the NHS and across partner organisations is essential. This is a matter for organisations, their Chief Executives, and their expert public health leadership.

50. **We will work with the Improvement & Development Agency, Modernisation Agency and**

the NHS Leadership Centre and the National College for School Leadership to identify the core skills and competencies that are needed for the new style of leadership that is required at different levels. This work will also recognise the development needs of managers and non-executives in PCTs and other health trusts, and will develop programmes that can be used to bring key players in local government and health together to plan action at a local level.

51. The creation of Primary Care Trusts created an important new focus for **public health** leadership, but has also stretched capacity. PCT Public Health Directors and their teams have a core role. Expert capacity is stretched and public health networks provide a way of sharing scarce resources as long as they are managed and supported. So SHAs should review the need to strengthen and develop networks to deliver the commitments in this White Paper.

52. SHA DsPH will oversee work with SHA workforce directorates, Regional Directors of Public Health, training directors and Deaneries to develop a robust local health improvement workforce plan to meet local needs. We will invest £5 million in 2005/06, and £30 million per annum from 2006/07 to support this work at a national and local level. This work will be assisted by the development of models to support local capacity and capability planning which encompass the whole workforce from health trainers to specialist practitioners. We will expect regional public health groups to play a key role in working with regional and local government to ensure adequate capacity to achieve local health improvement targets.

Summary

53. This adds up to a complex programme, with many contributors, locally, regionally and nationally.

54. Locally, the immediate focus will be the capacity planning that the NHS needs to begin with its

partners, to support Local Delivery Plans for 2005–06 to 2007–08. These will be followed by a National Workforce Strategy in spring 2005, which will have health improvement as an important component.

55. **We shall establish a Health Improvement Workforce Steering Group to develop a strategy and coordinate the action needed, within this framework, to ensure delivery of this White Paper.**

56. These actions will ensure that the drive for health improvement is integral to the NHS and supported by a strong infrastructure with the capacity and capability to deliver high quality health improvement services in partnership with other sectors.

SYSTEMS FOR LOCAL DELIVERY
The challenge

57. Along with the policies and goals we have described to improve health, we need to know what works and how to make this a reality across England. This section of the Annex describes and clarifies our concept of the system for these specific policies on health, concentrating on the NHS and local authority contributions. As part of our delivery plan we will ensure that everyone is clearer about who will do what, which organisations have the lead and our expectations of effective partnerships.

Introduction

58. In line with the Prime Minister's public sector reform principles, the overall direction, standards and values that guide the public sector elements of the system for improving health will be established nationally by agreement across Government. Devolution and delegation to the front line will give local leaders responsibility for delivery and the opportunity to design and develop services around the needs of local people.

59. This will be achieved by: aligning investment, performance assurance mechanisms, planning guidance, inspection and regulation processes to deliver increased flexibility; by reducing red tape; providing greater incentives and rewards for good performance; encouraging innovation; and enabling strong leadership and management at a local level.

Different organisations working together

60. Public sector contributions to delivering health at local level are not only through health structures, but also through local government. Alongside, and central to effective local delivery, are the contributions of independent businesses, voluntary organisations and the community sector, as well as individuals. This section of the Annex does not outline the contributions of sectors other than the NHS and local government. This will be addressed as part of the delivery plan.

61. The roles and responsibilities for individual NHS organisations originally outlined in the NHS Plan and Shifting the Balance of Power: Securing Delivery need to be fully adopted and consolidated throughout the NHS. Opportunities to support the health improvement agenda include joint appointments of Director of Public Health posts, utilisation of Health Act flexibilities, pooled budgets, integrated service teams and managed public health networks between PCTs and local authorities. The potential of these has not been fully realised. We will encourage PCTs to explore these and Strategic Health Authorities will be expected to empower and enable their NHS organisations to do so.

62. The NHS Improvement Plan signalled the need for major cultural change to address a shift from sickness to health. Cultural change is needed at all levels – both individual and corporate.

63. We need to be clear about the roles, responsibilities and accountabilities for organisations, partnerships and individuals.

We will establish coherence between planning processes, targets, incentives, performance measurement and inspection systems. As part of this process we will clarify the roles and responsibilities of public health specialists in the different parts of the system. Within the NHS we have already started to align these in ways that promote health through the recently issued NHS Improvement Plan and its supporting implementation programme, Improving the System. Where we have identified gaps, e.g. in the role of NHS Trusts and Foundation Trusts, we will issue additional guidance as part of the delivery plan for this White Paper.

64. Clinicians within the NHS will also need to address this cultural shift and view their individual roles and specialties within the context of improving health. All clinicians should enable patients to make healthier, more informed choices and ensure they are offered opportunities that will address prevention as well as treatment and care. We look to the professional bodies collectively to consider how they might ensure that this wider dimension to health care is addressed within the educational, training, development and regulatory frameworks for all clinical professionals.

65. We want to see an effective system for health delivered through close alignment between local community partners.

66. Supported by the existing and developing structural and organisational frameworks for NHS bodies, local authorities, networks and partnerships, this change will be sustained and reinforced throughout by alignment of:

- investment and resources;

- planning guidance and performance improvement regimes, including the balance between fewer nationally and more locally determined targets; and

- inspection, regulation and audit.

67. Structural and organisational arrangements have never delivered perfect alignment of resources and functions for the public sector. Wanless and the NHS Plan have confirmed that there is a sustainable institutional framework for the NHS, through which an effective system for health can be delivered that is closely aligned with local community partners.

68. In the NHS, Primary Care Trusts are population-based organisations which have a local focus, clear unequivocal responsibility for improving health. They have close contact with local leaders from other sectors, voluntary, business and local government, to deliver an integrated approach for their community.

69. Local authorities have responsibilities for social, economic and environmental wellbeing for their population as well as the duty of partnership with the NHS. Their contribution towards leadership of many local partnerships, and responsibility for health scrutiny place them alongside PCTs as the public sector leaders for addressing health inequalities, protecting the health of their local communities and promoting health to their populations.

70. The health improvement agenda for NHS Trusts, including Foundation Trusts, Care Trusts, etc is broadening. The national focus on health inequalities and health protection recognises the important role that NHS service providers have to play.

71. All types of NHS organisations, and particularly NHS Trusts and Foundation Trusts, must work with PCTs and other partners to contribute to health improvement in the local community, recognising their contribution to employment and economic development locally. The are expected to deliver these functions through the empowerment of clinical teams and patients, working across organisational and sectoral boundaries. They will encourage innovation and creativity in reaching out and providing services as close to local communities as possible, to maximise the benefit of NHS resources across the local community.

> Major contributions of Public Health professionals within NHS Trusts and other acute service providers are in relation to:
> - evidence-based clinical policy;
> - development of clinical governance;
> - high-quality information systems;
> - appraisal of health technology;
> - reduction of infection and health protection;
> - disease prevention;
> - pharmaco-epidemiology;
> - research;
> - green hospitals and the 'greening' of hospitals; and
> - the NHS as a corporate citizen.

72. The majority of NHS Arms Length Bodies contribute towards the system for public health and some have key responsibilities in the delivery of health improvement. Major examples are obviously the Healthcare Commission, which is described elsewhere in this Annex, but also the Health Protection Agency, NICE and the HDA. Other government agencies with key health improvement roles include the Environment Agency and the Food Standards Agency.

73. Health protection is a core component of an effective public health delivery system. Key national challenges such as influenza and SARs, uptake of immunisation, tuberculosis, sexual health including HIV/AIDS and chlamydia, infection control including MRSA and emergency preparedness are all important current challenges. The general public health infrastructure must be able to support delivery on these at a local level including the capacity for surge response in

emergencies. This requires robust relationships between the Health Protection Agency and the NHS with clarity around roles and responsibilities.

74. From April 2005 the Children Act 2004 places a duty on Strategic Health Authorities, Primary Care Trusts and others to cooperate with the local authority and its partners in making arrangements to improve the wellbeing of children. Wellbeing is defined in terms of the five outcomes of the Every Child Matters: Change for Children Programme: being healthy; staying safe; making a positive contribution; enjoying and achieving economic wellbeing.

Ways of working across boundaries: *partnerships and networks*

75. Partnership working has been referred to extensively and is key if local people are to get joined up and complementary services. An area-based (population) focus, rather than an organisation-based approach assists this.

76. At local level, the foundations of the public health system depend upon PCTs working closely with local authorities. Both work through key partnership mechanisms to develop and implement strategies, policies and plans to integrate, co-ordinate and develop services across both sectors.

77. Since 2001, Local Strategic Partnerships (LSPs) have provided some of the most important fora for partnership working on health. The best LSPs have been very effective in bringing about real improvement in the health of their community by facilitating joined-up planning and delivery.[1]

78. Alongside senior local government representation, leadership by Executive Officers of the NHS (eg Chief Executive) of both the PCT and engagement of senior representatives of other NHS organisations (eg Trusts) is often key to success.

79. Managed Public Health Networks provide a key mechanism to support the work of partnerships and organisations by providing highly specialised and essential public health skills, eg statistical analysis, health economics. PCTs, in partnership with their local NHS organisations and local authorities, should proactively manage specialist public health services and functions across the whole health community. Lessons should be learned from developing clinical networks, eg cancer, where investing in infrastructure, management, information, research and governance, as well as clinical leadership, has led to a step change in delivery.

80. Public Health Observatories (PHOs) are a key contributor towards partnerships and networks. An expanded role for public health observatories providing information to PCTs to inform locally commissioned services and providing local analysis and information to Local Government will build on the expertise of PHOs in the provision and assessment of regional data. PHOs will not replace the need for PCTs and local government to have their own information services, but will augment and complement this intelligence and knowledge network. PCTs will need to invest in PHOs to support this development.

81. In future, children's trusts will provide the focus for partnership working between health bodies, local authorities and other partners to improve the health of children and young people. This will encompass integrated strategy to develop a joint planning and commissioning strategy; integrated processes to involve health practitioners in utilising the common assessment framework and information sharing; and integrated front-line service delivery through multi-disciplinary teams and increasing co-location of health and other services.

---

1 Examples of best practice of local strategic partnerships working on health can be found in 'planning with a purpose' (http://www.hda.nhs.uk/Documents/planning_with_a_purpose.pdf) and 'pooling resources across sectors' (http://www.hda.nhs.uk/documents/poolingresources.pdf) and 'planning across LSPs' (http://www.hda-online.org.uk/downloads/pdfs/127805_NHS_TEXT.pdf)

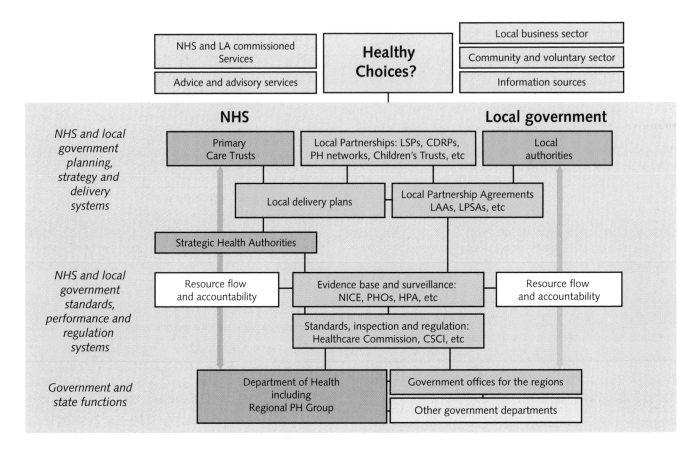

Strategic NHS and regional cross government oversight

82. Strategic Health Authorities are the headquarters for the local health economies of the NHS and are required to have specialist skills in public health. The responsibilities of SHAs are to ensure, through monitoring, improvement and management mechanisms, that the NHS is effectively delivering and contributing to improvements in health and reductions in inequalities in health. They also have a role with other NHS organisations to ensure effective delivery of health improvement, health protection and other public health functions (such as screening) to support delivery of this White Paper agenda.

83. The key role of the SHA will be to ensure that all organisations work together to improve health and reduce health inequalities. They will manage the performance of NHS programmes and networks that span organisational boundaries.

84. SHAs will support and develop PCTs and NHS Trusts to maximise their contribution to achieving the wider government agenda to improve health and wellbeing through local strategic partnerships. SHAs are expected to facilitate and empower, helping their NHS Trusts and PCTs to maximise their autonomy and develop a culture of health improvement and citizen involvement.

85. Government Offices were created in 1994, to bring together the activities and interests of different Government Departments in delivering Government policies in the English regions. In 2002/2003, Government Offices in the Regions (GORs) were responsible for around £9bn of Government expenditure. Their sponsor Departments are ODPM, Dept of Transport, DEFRA, DfES, DTI and the Home Office. They also act as host to co-located personnel from DCMS and DH.

Department of Health representatives located in the regions will:

- lead the work with regional and local government and the NHS to ensure that regional partner policies and activities take account of their health impact, eg housing, transport, planning, employment, education and skills, environment, rural affairs, crime and community safety;

- work in partnership with Strategic Health Authorities to ensure that the NHS contributes effectively to local partnerships such as LSPs and Crime and Disorder Reduction Partnerships and partnership agreements such as LAAs;

- lead the work with regional partners, including SHAs to bring together key performance processes to ensure there is cross-cutting analysis of delivery on health inequalities and joints support and drive processes;

- support SHAs to secure the NHS role in health improvement, particularly for NHS Trusts and Foundation trusts, in sustainable development frameworks across the regions and as an exemplar of social responsibility;

- lead the development and implementation of regional frameworks for health through work in partnership with regional assemblies, Government Offices and Regional Development Agencies;

- work with and through other relevant organisations, including the NHS and local authorities to implement national public health programmes within the region;

- contribute to the development and implementation of government policy; and

- ensure an effective regional intelligence and information function through the Public Health Observatories that supports the availability of regional and local information on health, for local people, the NHS, regional and local partners. This will include reports on health where requested by regional bodies.

86. The Department of Health has a well-established presence at regional level, under the leadership of the Regional Directors of Public Health (RDsPH). They provide leadership for the cross-government work on implementing policy on wider determinants of health in their regions and will oversee the performance of DH's cross government programmes and networks supporting wider determinants of health and reduction of inequalities.

87. Regional Directors of Public Health will have new responsibilities for ensuring that performance improvement information on cross-government agendas for wider determinants of health nationally, in Government Offices and other local and regional bodies, is communicated to and acted upon by Strategic Health Authorities and nationally.

88. A guide for the NHS on the roles and functions of regional partners in relation to health will be produced in 2005, highlighting how these individual partners contribute towards the overall delivery of an integrated cross-government approach to policy implementation for health and inequalities. Amongst others, this will address the role of the Regional Development Agencies, Regional Assemblies and their inter-relationships with the NHS.

Building leadership

89. All NHS organisations will need to lead for health if the NHS is to live out the commitments to health improvement, which form part of its founding purpose. So it is critical that there is adequate strategic leadership within the NHS and across partner organisations.

90. Other parts of the White Paper have already addressed issues relating to the general and specialist workforce for improving health, including public health professionals, and highlighted the need for leadership and leadership

development. This section of the annex looks specifically at supporting the corporate leadership culture across the NHS and local government to ensure a strengthened understanding of the corporate responsibility for improving health in all organisations.

91. We will target development for Chairs and Non-Executives in the NHS and Leaders and members in local government, together with their Chief Executives, Directors of Public Health, others at Board and Executive Director level, including those with professional leadership responsibilities.

92. These Corporate posts have important roles in:

   - providing focus and direction at local level;

   - giving visible and committed leadership;

   - demonstrating effective management for health;

   - demonstrating understanding of the principles affecting inequalities;

   - working in partnership; and

   - working to empower and inform local people and communities.

93. IDeA have pledged to contribute to the creation of a national workforce development strategy for improving health, including exploring the potential of bringing together NHS and local government leaders and managers for joint development opportunities. They will work with their counterparts within the NHS, the NHS Modernisation Agency leadership centre to secure these opportunities.

94. Critical to successful delivery of their responsibilities will be the influence and leadership of the local Director of Public Health. They will be expected to lead the PCTs' efforts to establish and maintain effective and close working relationships with local government, local partnerships and local

networks. We wish to underline our continuing commitment to the description of the local Director of Public Health contained in Shifting the Balance of Power: Securing Delivery. We also reinforce the need for significantly increased investment in capacity to support the delivery of the public health responsibilities supporting commissioning, service delivery and development and partnership working.

Ensuring local delivery

95. In the past, the NHS has been criticised for focusing too narrowly on its own immediate goals. The national cross Government Public Service Agreements and their targets and priorities can only be delivered through effective partnership working. It is important that standards, targets, incentives, support for change, planning, performance and inspection systems are aligned to encourage this. As a priority, this is essential between the NHS and local government, rather than focusing on individual organisations in isolation. Only by adopting this approach can we ensure coherence of delivery systems for health policies.

National standards

96. Recent guidance on standards, priorities and planning were brought together in the publication National Standards, Local Action, the Health & Social Care Standards & Planning Framework for 2005–06 to 2007–08. Improving health is identified as one of the four national priorities, with national targets to be met. Performance against standards are to be the main driver for continuous improvements in quality and will be assessed by the independent Healthcare Commission.

97. The standards refer to the need for systematic and managed disease prevention and health promotion programmes and has set action on health and inequalities firmly on the core agenda

for the NHS and its partners. Developing the NHS into a health service rather than one that focuses primarily on sickness is explicitly identified as a focus for the next stage of NHS reform.

98. Following publication of *National Standards, Local Action* the Department of Health issued a technical note to the NHS on Local Delivery Plans to support the delivery of these national targets. We will issue a supplementary technical note to the NHS, reinforcing the priorities of this White Paper and outlining the requirement to plan services to deliver reductions in health inequalities and improvements in obesity status, including among children, and on sexual health.

99. The LDP technical note already emphasises the need for plans to reduce inequalities, address cancer and coronary heart disease, reduce levels of smoking, improve infant mortality, reduce teenage conceptions and suicide mortality. The NHS is directed to develop plans for these national targets and priorities alongside the other national targets for access to services, MRSA, supporting people with long-term conditions and patient/user experience.

Aligning targets

100. The stretching national Public Service Agreements recently agreed with individual Departments have signalled the importance this Government attaches to improving health. The only national targets are those associated with the PSA, leaving greater flexibility for local organisations to determine how they should contribute to the delivery of national priorities.

101. PCTs have more headroom to set local targets in response to local needs and priorities. In developing targets in local plans, PCTs will be required to ensure that they are in line with population needs, address local service gaps, delivery equity, are evidence based, offer value for money and are developed in partnership with local

authorities. Partnership with local communities, service, providers, patients and service users and particularly with local authorities is highlighted as vital to ensuring that targets and commissioning plans are broadly based and not limited by individual organisational boundaries.

102. Recent changes in the relationships between central government and local delivery agencies within the public sector are already proving a spur to new initiatives and improvements in performance. In local government, the introduction of Local Public Service Agreements (LPSAs) add momentum to local partnerships. LPSAs are agreed between central government and local authorities and their partners, normally through the Local Strategic Partnership. Local partners select priorities for improvement locally and are paid a grant if they achieve targets agreed with central government (equal to around 2.5% of one year's expenditure, paid out in instalments over three years). The LPSA system offers a performance reward grant for achievement that motivates and focuses energy on the desired outcomes.

103. It is up to local partners to decide on the priorities. PCTs are expected to play an active part in helping define and support delivery of local action that benefits health – either directly or by addressing wider factors such as community safety or economic, environmental and social regeneration. So far, 36 upper-tier local authorities have set LPSA targets on health inequalities in the 'second generation' of negotiations, with many more on other areas of health. SHAs should work with regional public health groups to ensure that these are reflected in local target setting by PCTs.

104. The development of the Shared Priority between central and local government recognises the importance of healthy communities. This has led to CPA, the Pathfinder Programme, Beacon

Council scheme and Innovation Forum projects. The picture is larger than just agreeing Local PSAs.

105. For example, improvements in community safety, the educational performance of children, the skills of the workforce, the strength of the local economy and the cohesiveness and capacity of local communities all contribute to the well being and hence to the health of local people. These are not simply local authority priorities. From today they become priorities that the NHS shares. In the same way that the health service must address the wider determinants of health, local government must give a more explicit priority to health improvement, and must work to narrow health inequalities.

106. The more recent extension of this thinking has led to the government's proposals for pilot Local Area Agreements (LAAs). The level of response to the invitation to seek pilot status demonstrated the high level of support for this approach. A significant motivating factor behind LAAs is the promise that separate local funding streams will be merged to give greater flexibility to local authorities and their partners. The themes within LAAs have significant relevance to health.

Incentives

107. Funding is available to support increased investment in the NHS. By 2007–08, total investment in the NHS will rise to £90 billion. Primary Care Trusts will control over 80% of this. They are able to direct an increasing proportion towards local priorities for action and to improve the health of their communities. Nationally, Government will support their efforts through increased investment in campaigns, in research and evaluation, and in information systems.

108. We need the right incentives – for individuals, clinicians, other employees and organisations – to put health first. The coherent system of national and local targets, assessment arrangements and

inspections spanning the NHS and local Government now creates a strong overall framework for this and is described in more detail next. More is needed to redress the NHS's traditional focus and to rebalance investment in favour of sustainable health and healthcare systems.

Support for change

109. The Government recognises that the strength of public interest in the Choosing Health? consultation reflects a strong expectation that there will be changes in our traditional approaches to service planning and delivery. The challenge to the public sector is not just to do new things, but to do them in new ways which engage with individuals, communities and other organisations and businesses to deliver sustainable improvements in the health of the whole population, and a narrowing of the health gap that exists between different groups and communities. In short, we need a culture change programme across large parts of the public sector.

110. For the NHS, supporting the implementation phase of the Public Health White Paper will be a priority task for the NHS Modernisation Agency (MA) and for the national body that will replace the Modernisation Agency from April 2005. It will work alongside PCTs, SHAs and DH to achieve this by focusing on how change can be achieved and embedded across local communities and the health and government system.

111. Implementation rests with local organisations, their communities and individuals. The MA will contribute leading edge improvement expertise, best practice tools, techniques and strategies for change so that the potential for effective and lasting change is enhanced.

112. Innovation processes will be built into implementation and creative ideas can be generated. It will help to test the applicability

There is a nationally agreed general medical services (GMS) contract, used by 60% of general practice. Practices are obliged to provide *essential* services for those who are ill or believe themselves to be ill, and chronic disease management and appropriate health promotion. Nearly every practice offers *additional* services, such as flu jabs, cervical smears and maternity medical services. Many practices also offer *enhanced* services, often provided by a practitioner with a special interest, such as drug abuse services, specialised sexual health services or diagnostics.

- **Personal medical services (PMS)** are a more locally sensitive model, where a contract is agreed with the PCT. PMS contractors may also provide quite specialised services in primary care settings.
- Where it is agreed locally to be necessary, the PCT itself can directly provide services. For example, it might directly employ a GP or a care manager to support the care of those people with many health problems.

- Finally, through **alternative provider medical services**, a PCT can contract for provision of any necessary care for its population, with the private, voluntary or charitable sectors, alone or in partnership with each other or other NHS providers.
- All contracting routes will offer well-organised care that can be monitored through the Quality and Outcomes Framework and over 95% of practices do so. This is an incentivised scheme where there are a number of standards of quality care, other indicators of the way care can be well-organised, access standards and patient experience questionnaires.
- The proposed new pharmacy contract will reflect the public health role of pharmacists both within the essential services component of the contract, which all pharmacists will normally provide, and the locally commissioned enhanced services, which PCTs will commission *essential services* and *enhanced services* to meet local need.

of proven healthcare improvement methods in a wider health context. It will support the identification of best practice changes that have the highest impact, assessing the potential benefits of these changes and the gains that local communities and organisations can make as a result.

113. The ambitious goals of the Public Health White Paper require fresh and innovative perspectives on how to create large-scale change across an entire county. Planned and programmed approaches to change need to be combined with actions to ignite energy and passion around the cause of health, rather than illness, and in doing so, create a locally led, grass roots movement. We will help to support the continued development of the movement for health and well being.

114. The Improvement and Development Agency has pledged to contribute towards the delivery of the national objectives within the White Paper. IDeA and the Local Government Association both endorse recognition the key role of local government in improving health and promoting well being of local communities and have pledged to help drive this agenda forward through their work. To support this, they will pay particular attention to developing greater awareness of health inequalities and the potential contribution of local government to their reduction. Local Councillors will be supported to develop their roles as community leaders for changes that will increase the opportunity for local people to adopt healthier lifestyles and provide environments that protect their communities.

115. We, together with the NHS Modernisation Agency, have recruited ten Regional Change Advisers. They will focus on supporting the change programme which local authorities, Primary Care Trusts and other local partners will be developing in pursuit of their new duty in the Children Bill to make arrangements for local cooperation. This will involve support in moving towards children's trusts to deliver better outcomes for children and young people and in implementing the National Service Framework for Children, Young People and Maternity Services. As part of this agenda, the Regional Change Advisers will support Primary Care Trusts and Strategic Health Authorities in taking forward the actions in this White Paper.

Inspection and performance assessment

116. From 2005 there will be a new performance framework for the NHS and social care, described in *Standards for Better Health*. This set out the level of quality all organisations providing NHS care will be expected to meet or aspire to across the NHS in England. One of the seven domains in *Standards for Better Health* is public health.

117. The independent Healthcare Commission is responsible for developing assessment criteria to be used to determine whether core standards have been met, and judging progress against developmental standards. The annual performance ratings will be based on annual reviews of NHS organisations and those providing services to the NHS and will draw on thematic reviews of particular functions and services, including those for health improvement and public health.

118. In parallel the Audit Commission uses the Comprehensive Performance Assessment (CPA) methodology to assess local authority performance, focusing particularly on continuous improvement, outcomes for service users, proportionality to performance and risk, and partnership. The CPA methodology is being revised for 2005, with development work underway. Assessment of Councils' performance in promoting healthy communities and narrowing health inequalities will be a key part of the new Comprehensive Performance Assessment framework from 2005.

119. The Healthcare Commission and Audit Commission have agreed to work together on the way in which these new systems assess health improvement. In their combined response to the Choosing Health? Consultation they proposed a several stranded approach to joint work on assessing health improvement and public health on the basis that ' regulation has its part to play in improving (public) health and the regulators must also work in partnership to be effective' The specific proposals include:

'The Healthcare Commission and Audit Commission will seek to align their approaches to assessment of local government and healthcare organisations to produce a common locality based view of progress and performance in improving population health and reducing health inequalities. These will also need to take account the context set by the relevant regional and sub regional bodies.

'The Healthcare Commission and the Audit Commission will develop a framework for thematic reviews of public health issues to inform national and local delivery. Other inspectorates will be involved wherever appropriate.'

120. From 2005, there will also be a single overall inspection framework for children, to underpin all relevant inspections carried out by the Healthcare Commission, the Commission for Social Care Inspection, Ofsted, the Audit Commission and others. This will focus on how services contribute to the overall wellbeing of children and young people, including their physical and mental health. Joint area reviews will look at how children's services are working together to this end.

Summary

121. The systematic approach for delivering improvements in health at a local level will depend on:

   ▪ Strong leadership and management

   ▪ Commitment to working effectively in partnership

   ▪ Aligned inspection and regulation, standards, targets, incentives and performance assurance mechanisms

Making a difference

122. This time we have to build and sustain public health action across Government and at all other levels. A robust delivery system will integrate and develop this systematic approach to deliver the new public health agenda. The White Paper spells out the key challenges for Government, establishing health as a way of life for individuals and communities. This requires us to build effective partnerships and invest to ensure future health and take effective action to reduce inequalities. Health is inextricably linked to the way in which people live their lives, so only if we consider health as an integral part of policy development and implementation at national and local level will we achieve our aim to improve England's health.

Printed in the UK for The Stationery Office Limited
on behalf of the Controller of Her Majesty's Stationery Office
174559   11/04

२५